DON'T LOSE OUT, WORK OUT

DON'T LOSE OUT, WORKOUT

RUJUTA DIWEKAR

First published by Westland Publications Private Limited in 2014

Published by Westland Books, a division of Nasadiya Technologies Private Limited, in 2022

No. 269/2B, First Floor, 'Irai Arul', Vimalraj Street, Nethaji Nagar, Alapakkam Main Road, Maduravoyal, Chennai 600095

Westland and the Westland logo are the trademarks of Nasadiya Technologies Private Limited, or its affiliates.

ISBN: 9789395073097

10 9 8 7 6 5 4 3

Typeset by Ram Das Lal, New Delhi, NCR

Printed at Thomson Press (India) Ltd

Contents

Prologue

Don't Lose Out

'Maut aur tatti kabhi bhi aa sakti hai,' said Javed, my guide on the Kolahoi glacier trek in Kashmir, as he quickly ran behind a rock. 'The most astonishing fact about human beings is that we all live as if we are going to live forever,' said dharmaraj Yudhishthir, and won the life of his 4 brothers in return, goes a story in the *Mahabharat*. 'Life is but a pause between the first breath and the last.' 'The only thing you can guarantee at somebody's birth is his or her death, everything else is unpredictable.'

I am sure that, like me, you have heard and read endless stories and theories and researches on death and life after death. However, all we have access to is our life in its current form and what we do with it. And every moment of our life we are subjected to catabolism, the technical term for breakdown or destruction of our cells. And though we remain fascinated with death and theories around it, we remain quite indifferent to the process of catabolism that is happening in the body even as you read this. Catabolism can even be called preparation for physical death, but let's make it more accessible to what we are ready to understand and call it the process of ageing. Now all those who wanna age quickly put your hands up, and all those who want to delay it go answer the doorbell. What's this, no hands are going up and nobody is going to answer the door either? Listen, one of the things you can do to reduce catabolism is get more active in daily life. Small activities help in a large way to arrest ageing and the associated deterioration in our jnanedriyas and karmendriyas, but the lion's share lies with regular physical exercise.

Metabolism = break down + build up

Let me explain — life blesses us with anabolism, the ability to build our bodily cells (and also our habits, beliefs, character, destiny and our workout routine). According to exercise or sports science, anabolism and catabolism, the process of building up and breakdown, together make for metabolism, our body's daily energy or calorie expenditure. The Greek root of the word metabolism is *metabole,* which means to change, and metabolism does keep changing during our lifetime; the longer time you spend on earth, the lower your metabolism gets. There are many reasons for this, the main one being that you get progressively fat, fatter, who knows currently you may even be at your fattest. Not just that, your fat free mass (bones, muscles, etc.), gets less and less. Why, you ask. Well don't ask me, evolution built in this process of loss of lean tissue and gain in fat mass to ensure that there is no 'overcrowding', matlab to ensure that you die and don't occupy space meant for your offspring. So grandfather marne ke baad bedroom becomes available for the grandchild, get it?

Some of the ways in which ageing occurs are:

1. Skeleto–muscular changes

Ok, I said this before and I want to say this again, we get progressively fatter and start losing out on our muscle or body tone, i.e. lose out on our lean tissue. The size of our muscle cell, or what is technically called as the cross-section of our muscle fibre, reduces or goes through atrophy (shrinkage), while the size of the fat cell increases. This process leads to a change in not just our total body weight but also in factors that contribute to our body weight. Now, more than ever, our fat mass seems to contribute to this magical body weight number, and, largely, till you get to around 80 +, the number is likely to grow. Post that, there will be an even accelerated atrophy of the bone, muscle and the fat tissue and you are likely to get skinny and will start rapidly losing your strength. The changes don't occur at once, they happen phursat mein, in slow mo. They kind of start once we are in our 30s, accelerate towards our menopause or andropause and then it's a slippery slope from there on. We seem to lose more strength and gain more fat on our lower body first, our legs lose out on strength faster than our hands and we collect more girth around our hips, stomach and thighs. According to me, this happens because, typically, as we get older and richer, the less we want to use our legs. We won't walk, take the bus or run for the train, or for that matter won't even open the door, draw our curtains or walk to the kitchen to get a glass of water. In India, the richer you get the less physical activity you are supposed to do to help yourself, it's not passed by the Constitution but we live by this like a law.

Can you do something about it? Of course you can, but we will come to that later. For now let's look at what's happening to the bones. Our bone mineral density goes down and our bone matrix starts getting weaker. Our bones are made up of minerals, the most important of them being calcium. Up to 4% of our total body weight comes from mineral weight and this weight starts going down. So let's say you weighed 50 kg when you were 25 years old, then around 2 kg is the contribution from mineral weight. Now you are 50 years old and 75 kg, the contribution from mineral weight will not be 3 kg, in fact if you have gone through the regular sedentary lifestyle it may be much less than 2 kg.

Hope you are getting my point of how **contribution of lean body weight to total body weight decreases and therefore we feel less strong**, or less able to support our own body weight. The bone matrix (think of this like a spiral fishing net kind of structure, in the holes of which minerals like calcium deposit themselves to form a strong dense bone) starts weakening, almost like a torn fishing net, and our bones, joints, tendons and ligaments start struggling to support our own body weight. Most of the time there is an oedema or swelling, as fluid starts getting collected around our joints, again first in the weight-bearing joints, as the ankles and knees take the max toll. A small slip or fall leads to a fracture and many of us have lost our grandmothers to a hip fracture that led to bed rest and eventually to death.

2. Hormonal changes

Yes, they change, estrogen and testosterone levels drop and you don't need me to tell you this, but one of the major changes is in the insulin sensitivity. Insulin is supposed to be an anabolic hormone, that which helps the body grow, and as this hormone starts getting sluggish, our cells start feeling starved for their daily dose of nutrients, and that's exactly how diabetes makes the grand entry into our lives.

Yes, this is supposed to happen at a more 'mature' age, 50+, but as our cars / internet connection / lives get faster and our bodies get slower, we see this as early as 25. No wonder then that chronological age gets more and more irrelevant and biological age, both the term and its meaning, is what really matters.

3. All the involuntary systems change

Our heart, lungs, digestive system also 'age', which means that they perform less effectively under the same workload. For example: you eat 2 wada pavs at 6 p.m. in college, you don't remember it at 6 the next morning. As a company executive, when you look at a wada pav at 6 p.m. after a sales meeting, all you think about is your haalat on the pot the next morning. Basically you have a heart and stomach for less adventure, less risk and less food.

Exercise to the rescue

Chalo, I can write endlessly about ageing — what I have written about is only the tip of the iceberg. The main reason why I even thought of including this section in the book is because **every Indian has a burning desire to live or die without being a burden** (financial or emotional) on their children or immediate family members. We want to die 'haste haste' or after a meal or in our sleep and of course we want to play with grandchildren before that. But we live doing nothing about fulfilling this desire. We condemn spending money on gyms, indulge in morning walks more for fun than for fitness, have long gaps between our meals, sleep with the TV on, basically make very little time or monetary investment into ensuring that disability, partial or total, will not occur. And this needs to change, because a well-structured exercise plan can do miracles, really. It can reverse ageing or anti-age us by as much as 20 years in as little as 12 weeks. Which means, take that wheelchair away, aunty ji is now gonna walk ulta on the escalator.

Before we dive deeper into the technicalities of exercise, let's get a few things clear in our head:

a) A journey of 1000 miles starts but with one small step: If you feel that you have wasted a lot of time, then do me a favour, don't spend a second more on thinking about when you should have started your exercise program or how you shouldn't have quit basketball / tennis or whatever after Std 10. Just start exercising; that one day that you begin is a stepping stone to the lifelong commitment that you need for exercise.

b) Something is better than everything: Yeah, don't fall into that trap of 'will start post Diwali / weekend / exam / presentation', so that you can be 'regular'. Being regular is always a challenge and you will need to work at that continuously. Starting a month, day or year later will not make it any easier, it will only make it more difficult. And with exercise, working out 3 days in this month is better than working out every alternate day next month because this whole 'next month' thing is only a fantasy.

By the way, you are not alone, everybody, every single person feels like exercising 'tomorrow'. When I was in China for the Indo-China yoga and health summit, the legendary BKS Iyengar said, 'Every day I feel I will do yoga tomorrow, not today.' So don't blame yourself for feeling like that. If the 95-year-old who took to yoga at the age of 7 or 8 and has been at it daily since then can feel that, then we are only human.

c) Training costs money, so be prepared to pay: Hey! Training costs money, seriously. So just change your mindset: instead of being prepared to pay 'everything to save yourself or your loved one', just pay a little bit every month, to your trainer / gym membership / yoga class, etc., and save your wealth by ensuring good health.

The brain is pre-programmed / likes short-term awards

My guide Javed told me fascinating stories about the strife in Kashmir while walking up with me to Kolahoi glacier in Lidder valley. He had immense respect for the Indian army and believed that Kashmir would always be let down by the governments, be it at the Centre or the State. Politics, he professed, was the same everywhere and politicians by jaat are harami. The army, he said, was like the aam Kashmiri, getting crushed between Centre and State, but like the Kashmiri, the army is dil ka saaf and jabaan ka pucca.

Seeing my surprise at this statement, he then went on to narrate an incident that had taken place a few years ago when he was travelling as a horseman with some yatris on the way to Amarnath. At Chandanwari, the base camp, there was random firing in the night by terrorists, and 6 people inside Javed's tent died. Only Javed and his friend, another horseman, survived; stroke of luck, he said. The next thing they know, some officers from the Indian army barged into the tent to inspect what had happened, and on finding 6 dead bodies, one of the officers hit Javed's head with the butt of his gun. His ear bled all night. The next morning Javed went to the army camp, ear still bleeding, and complained to the 'bada sahib'.

The bada sahib said, ok, I will punish the guy who did this to you. The soldier who had hit Javed was made to stand in dhoop with his gun raised over his head for 3 hours. If he lowered his arms even for a minute, an hour was to be added to his punishment. Instant punishment and knowing whom to trust is what made the Indian army the hero for Javed and all other horsemen on that journey. 'He will now think before he raises his gun,' Javed winked. Compared to the humiliation he faced and the wound still visible on the side of his ear, a 3-hour punishment to stand in the sun with a gun raised hardly seems 'fair', but the fact that there was an instant response was the deciding factor for him.

I feel it's exactly this part of the brain that gets used in most weight loss / exercise plans. You get people to work hard and promise a 'reward' that is not tangible or seen or recognized like better flexibility, ability to run faster, lift heavier weights, etc., and it doesn't hook the audience as much. But currents on a machine, 15 minutes in the steam and an almost zero-calorie diet with the 'reward' of a 100g lost almost every single day on the weighing scale does the trick. The brightest and smartest people who would otherwise recognize that this is just water weight lost and the fat is not moving seem to fall for this reward system. It's because the brain is pre-programmed for the instant reward / punishment thing. That's also the reason why people want that pastry at that very instant; even if it makes them feel terrible for hours later, the fact that at that moment it rewards, does it for them.

It's important to understand this aspect of the brain when

you commit to a fitness journey. It's your body after all, and not some game you are playing where you need an instant reward / punishment system in place. A real change in your fitness levels takes time and is 100 times more rewarding, meaningful and sustainable than 100g lost on the scale.

How exercise anti-ages

Every time you work out, your body goes through microscopic breakdown, a catabolic reaction. The muscular tissue which has gone through breakdown is then repaired by the body (anabolism), the process is called adaptation, and if your body is convinced that you are going to be regular at exercise, then it ensures that it repairs and rebuilds enough tissue so that the next time you work out at the same load or training intensity, no breakdown will be caused. This leads to **hypertrophy or increase in the muscle tissue**, and builds density in the bones, reversing the very process of ageing. **In short, working out is a catabolic process that promotes anabolism.** As long as you are working out at the right intensity, the anabolism process or the calories required for the repair, rebuilding and maintenance processes will be much more than the catabolic process. So you will be reversing the process of breakdown or ageing in the body by proving to your body's intelligence that you are using your muscles so it should not lose them or break them down or go through atrophy.

Will all this also lead to weight loss? What do you think? Of course. For one, working out itself is a calorie-burning process, then the repair, rebuilding process is another calorie burner and this process takes up to 48 hours at times, which means you burn more calories for 2 days post a workout session (you will learn details later in the book). And to top it all, because your workout changes your body composition or ensures that you have more muscle as compared to fat, it accelerates your basal metabolism too. Without working out, a sedentary lifestyle will cause you to have more fat than muscle and will decrease your BMR. Because **fat is an inert tissue, it doesn't demand calories from your body to maintain itself**, it is easier for your body to keep it vs. keeping muscle.

The other things that can put you in an anabolic zone are:

A good eating plan: Read *Don't Lose Your Mind, Lose Your Weight*. When you are on a low cal / low fat / low whatever diet, you breakdown much more in your body than your ability to build up, you feel so low on energy, you can't even think of gymming or lifting your hand to straighten your hair, result — ageing and accelerated ageing because of fat deposition. A diet that is high on nutrients makes you feel in the zone to exercise. When you exercise you break down yes, but building up processes cost more than break down, result — fat loss + younger skin, hair, face and waist.

Good quality sleep: Read *Women & the Weight Loss Tamasha* for details. An irregular bedtime is the biggest contributor to skipping exercise. Not just that, all the anabolic hormones (those which help your body repair, rebuild, maintain, etc.) surge in the night. With poor quality sleep, you don't have enough anabolic hormones like growth hormone etc., and it results in a fatter and older you.

Healthy relationships: Come on, have a stressful boss or an unstable partner and you will age quickly. But if you are 'boring' enough to have found your calling early in life both on the personal and professional fronts, then your catabolism or breakdown process stays low and your anabolic or 'happy states' dominate. So there you go, don't like the wrinkles under your eyes, blame your spouse;-).

The exercise high

'Ok, now even I can tell you something "abnormal"' smiled Smrithi, my friend from Darjeeling who belongs to the Limbu tribe, on learning that I, and all of us from Konkan, believe in ghosts, and that my grand-uncle's rationale was if I existed, so did the ghosts. 'You know after 5 days of the death of a loved one, we sacrifice a boar and throw a party where all the grieving members of the family sing and dance.' I winked and giggled and exclaimed, 'Get up and move on with life, nice strategy.' The sacrifice of an animal is common amongst some tribes in India, but the dancing intrigued me and suddenly a neuron jumped in my brain and said — 'the runner's high'. The runner's high is actually both gym and lab lingo for the rise in 'feel good' chemicals in the brain. Depression or feeling low is marked by a decrease in serotonin and norepinephrine, and exercise (or dancing, like in Smrithi's tribe's case) increases the exact same neurotransmitters. So you can actually work out or dance your way out of depression and sadness. Studies have shown that exercise is actually much more effective than anti-depressants as a form of therapy, with you looking better as the only side effect ☺.

But forget all that, learn this, **more catabolism than anabolism = fat deposition**. Which means that if the catabolic component of metabolism is higher than the anabolic component then there is an increase in the body fat stores. And the only thing that you can do in your daily life to ensure that there is a big surge in the calories or energy required by anabolism, is work out and work out at an intensity that is respectful. In short, don't crawl when you can walk. The other side of this equation, the positive side, is if anabolism is more than catabolism, what will be burned darling, or where will be the deficiency be compensated from? Fat tissue again. So know that you are right when you don't trust those creams or surgical procedures for anti-ageing, they can't reverse ageing, coz they increase catabolism and decrease anabolism. **The only way out is working out, the only legal, sensible, sustainable way to increase anabolism and to anti-age.**

A short note for readers

I have been carrying this book in my stomach for as long as I can remember, perhaps from the time that I started working as a 'warm up instructor', someone who would assist the main instructor in an aerobic class, during my undergrad days as an Ind. Chemistry student. In 1999, I finished my PG in Sports Science and Nutrition and completed the first step towards 'formal education' in fitness. Very few people would have my kind of qualification, a degree to back and hands-on experience, but what I noticed is that to give advice on fitness, weight loss and exercise, you actually needed none. Everyone I met everywhere, was a pro. Everyone would speak on exercise with authority and finesse. People who couldn't tell their pyruvic from lactic, their myoglobin from haemoglobin, their Type 1 from Type 2, were experts. Experts because they, well, spoke like they had expertise in the field. So I really needn't have bothered with formal education but my mother said that just graduation would reflect poorly on her, so I had to have a MINIMUM of post grad and later, as long as I was educated, she had no problem whether I became a 'fitness expert' or a 'plumbing expert'.

Earlier in my career my response to statements like 'gymming makes you bulky', 'running kills your knees', 'forward bends are to be avoided after a slip disc', etc., would be lamba chauda bhashans. Passionate ones, filled with more anger than facts, more disgust than reason, more talking, less listening. Then it occurred to me that first and foremost, I need to behave like a professional. Bole toh, not open my mouth till there's money on the table. That, if I said the same things but in return for money, they would mean something to people, otherwise it was just garam hava. That people are always going to turn around and say 'but there is so much conflicting information' and the reason why there was conflicting information is because they were listening to everyone, and in the same vein they would listen to me. Money would mean that they would listen to me over everyone else, and if I had to get people to value my advice, then I would have to learn to value it first. Essentially not give it out on impulse or because I happen to overhear something but because I got paid to talk. In exchange for money, I would buy their sincerity and an honest attempt to follow the advice. My job would be quite simple then, educate, update, practice and give out the most honest advice based on what I know. And immediately it set me free from the complication or complexity of thinking that my job was to convince people: it wasn't, it was to give honest advice.

Today of course, shutting up has become an integral part of my job. When runners look down upon others simply because they don't run, bulky arms with skinny calves look down upon the treadmill, yoga addicts close eyes and do pranayama in trains and gardens, I realize that it is not entirely funny and mostly it is the way it is because of mis-information, or shall I say half-information. And half-information is a dangerous thing, especially when it concerns your health and wellbeing.

This book then is an attempt to turn the half information on exercise to complete information, things we should have been taught in school (along with nutrition) with the same seriousness as any other science, because how fit and unfit we stay influences the lives we lead and how complete or fulfilling they are.

And I do sincerely hope that you will like what you read and that it will give new direction and meaning to your efforts to exercise. And yes, thanks for buying the book, when you could have gotten exercise advice for free from anywhere ☺.

Rujuta Diwekar
Mumbai
November 2013

Chapter 1

Exercise Myths

There is this thing about myths. The longer they're around, the closer they migrate to becoming facts. People swear by them, they will give examples of 'someone' they know who has benefited or lost weight or managed some such 'result'. Sometimes they even get attached to these myths like they would to their loved ones and are offended if someone even raises a doubt. But the fact remains that myths are what they are — misinterpretations, misunderstandings and oversimplifications. So let's look at some of the most common exercise myths, understand why they exist and learn why you should not believe what 'they say'.

Spot reduction — the mother of all myths

Once upon a time in Mumbai, many years ago, as I was climbing down the stairs to the gym in the basement (ever wondered why the most posh clubs and hotels have gyms in the basement?), I saw Jaspal smiling at my reflection in the mirror. Half his smile was pride, the other half was pain. He was groaning as he beat his knees into his flabby, podgy stomach. 'Jaspal, STOP!' I screamed. 'What are you doing?' And like a flash of lightning it hit me — he was trying to pummel his stomach in. His pride arose from the fact that he was putting his body through unbearable pain, that he was ready to do 'anything' to lose his paunch. 'God, Jaspal! Stop!' I heard myself say again.

'They say if you cycle with your knees hitting the stomach, it will reduce.' 'Pagal! They are pagal,' I shouted. Jaspal looked confused; I was his trainer, I should be happy, and that's exactly what he said, 'You should be HAPPY. I cycled like this for twenty minutes.'

You may not have met Jaspal or encountered his close-to-suicidal attempt at reducing his stomach, but you must have met Mrs Khanna who does 500 crunches every day for a flat stomach, or apne gym ke official broker, Patel uncle, who puts a stick on his shoulders, à la herdsmen style, and then revolves around his own axis to get rid of his 'sides'. Mrs Khanna gets to keep her stomach, Patel uncle keeps his sides, all that both lose is some precious time. You smarty-pants got what I am hinting at? Spot reduction is all garam hava. Yeah, that's exactly what it is. Both Patel and Khanna are more likely to pass gas during their workout than burn any fat from the stomach or sides or whatever.

Chalo, everything said and done, Patel made 20 khoka on his gold stocks and Mrs Khanna's kids are school toppers, so these two aren't exactly dumb, gas-passing idiots. Then why do they indulge in these activities? Very simply, because they didn't think exercise is an important enough subject to understand deeply or because this book wasn't written earlier (come on allow me some self-indulgence, wink wink).

Why does this myth exist?

Just like the term movement goes with bowel, the term burn goes with fat. So everybody is trying to 'burn' fat, and is told that one of the best ways to experience the 'burn' is crunches, side kicks, leg lifts, etc. Iske kai saare fayde hai — for example, it requires no equipment, so simply give some lying down space to the fat aunty or give the space in front of the mirror to the enthu uncle and they will pay gym membership for an entire year without even once using a single piece of equipment.

Ok, I will tell you the REAL reason: when you contract your muscle endlessly — the rectus abdominus in crunches or the abductor in the side kicks — they produce a by-product of muscular contraction called lactic acid. Now this lactic acid is what gives you the BURN, and really has nothing to do with the fat on top of the muscle. In fact, the main difference between muscle and fat tissue is that muscle has the property to contract and relax while fat has the property to sag, it can neither contract nor relax. Exercise physiologists call it the 'non-working entity' of the human body. So when you lift your legs up or chest and shoulders off the floor, **the fat just sits there enjoying the joy ride**, the muscle overworks and produces tons of lactic acid, begging your brain to stop this voluntary contraction / torture.

Yes, that's exactly why the human body produces lactic acid. If the concentration of lactic acid increases beyond an acceptable limit, then the brain gets the signal to stop the activity. Lactic acid creates a steadily increasing burn that produces a peculiar pain and the brain is wired to ask the muscles to stop the contraction (self-induced) so that the burn or pain can be stopped.

Now, is the human brain stupid to stop the body from 'fat burning'? Of course not. It is rooted in reality and logic and knows that the production of lactic acid beyond an acceptable limit means that the muscle is being overworked. If the muscle is getting overworked, then the ligament, tendon, joint and bone around which this over-enthu contraction is being carried out will soon be at risk of snapping, pulling, breaking. Oops, oops, can't allow that. This is after all an exercise to make the body — including the bones, tendons, ligaments, joints — stronger, not weaker or vulnerable to injury.

Sadly, we understand exercise so little, that just as your brain asks you to stop, your trainer says, 'One more, come on one more, feel that burn, let that fat melt, come on, don't give up now.' And as the good sense of the brain finally takes over you crash land to the floor, feeling like a fool with no will power to burn fat and therefore doomed to stay fat. And your trainer just smirks, 'No pain, no gain.'

So should you not do crunches or leg lifts or work your sides? Of course you should. But it can't be the only thing you do in the gym. It can't even be a priority exercise if fat loss is on your mind (details in Chapters 2 and 3). But you can definitely do 2 or 3 sets of 10-15 reps once in a week or 2 weeks. That way it will serve the purpose of moving muscles in that specific angle and not overload your joints or your gym time.

Running is bad for the knees

OR — Running? Are you mad? Knee replacement ka irada hai?

'Don't run, it will harm your knees,' these were the last words of the kala kutta who peed with regularity on your car tyres outside Joggers' Park. Bad joke, I agree. But really, everybody seems to tell you or rather warn / scare / threaten you with dire consequences if you so much as talk about running. So how do all these people who don't run know about the ill-effects of running?

The logic that is at work here is the same wherein everybody who's not married knows about the many benefits of being married. Married people, on the other hand, know that it's not marriage but how you approach marriage that decides your happiness quotient and have also understood that getting married is rather risky if you are not fully prepared for the inevitable change in equations.

So as marriage changes equations between people and the crux of a good marriage lies in having equal ownership of responsibilities and resources, running changes the equation between your feet and the ground and good running would require that the body weight and the forces that it exerts are equally distributed along your weight-bearing joints.

Anyway public, to cut a long story short, if you are really seeking running advice, listen to a runner, not to a doctor or the liftman or to that kala kutta, unless of course they are runners themselves.

But do people actually risk getting knee injuries while running? Of course, just like you risk becoming plain bored by getting married. So are you doomed? No. You simply need to understand the biomechanics of running and free yourself from this risk. Running has something called a 'non-contact phase', where both your feet are off the ground. So when you land, the foot that strikes the ground lands with more than 4 to 6 times your body weight. If you haven't spent time strengthening the muscles around your thigh or stretched them, then you are risking an injury not so much because you ran, but because you gave your running very little thought.

Stretching and strengthening the muscles involved in running is crucial; without adequate strength and flexibility, you would injure your knee even if you were not running and just 'brisk walking' or even channel surfing. The only difference is that, with walking, you would injure it in 2 years instead of 2 months. And then of course you wonder what happened. You were so regular with 'exercise'. Really? You were just regular with abuse. Exercise means indulging in activity after proper thought and analysis; if you did all that, you would be stretching and strengthening too. Just like marriage gets boring, running leads to knee injury because, instead of spending time on wholesome aspects of running like stretching and strengthening, you spent time buying yellow shoes and matching tracks. Very much like how you forgot to look at your wife when she said something important and focused on buying her the latest iPhone.

Corollary — Don't walk on the treadmill, it will ruin your back

So everyone wants us to live long, stay slim and will even say that walking is the 'best exercise', but warn you about back problems if you walk on the treadmill. But your main problem is that you can ONLY walk on the treadmill and have no time to go to the beach or park for a walk. Listen, just read the earlier myth again. Walking on the treadmill / running will kill the back (or knee, ankle, hip — all weight-bearing joints) only if you don't invest in stretching and strengthening the muscles around these joints. But if I have already said that earlier, why am I saying it again and wasting paper when you are all for saving trees? Ok, it's because I have a specific point to make about treadmills. Only walk or run on the treadmill at a speed at which you can comfortably do so without having to hold the side bars or the front panel. If you burned '500 kcals' or ran at '9.5' or walked for '1 hour' but did so by resting your weight on one of the treadmill's many branches, then you essentially taxed your back (or the most vulnerable weight-bearing joint in your body) and ensured that some orthopaedic somewhere, struggling to meet his target of x number of surgeries to continue operating at the 5-star hospital, just found his bakra.

So when it comes to running on the treadmill, learn to hold your body weight first, and learn to run without load-shedding on the treadmill, and your back will be safe. Not just safe but even stronger. Remember, technique matters more than number of calories.

If you weight train you will get bulky

Yeah and if you go to the loo you will pee. Arre, the very idea of going to the gym is to bulk up; technically it's called hypertrophy or growth of the muscles. Muscles, as you know, are the fat-burning furnaces of the body, and when you grow muscle you grow your body's ability to sport a flat stomach and a tight butt — now who wouldn't like that? Everybody would, but everybody is scared of looking like a 'body builder', or in the case of women, looking like a 'man'. Now first things first, nobody looks like a body builder because they simply went to the gym. I mean it's no matter of chance, it's a matter of devotion, blood, sweat, guts and sacrifice. People who want to look like 'builders' work hard to do so and most times fail. So even before you start thinking about gymming, rid yourself of this irrational fear.

Now don't get me wrong, I know what you mean, you

don't want to look disproportionately bulky, or in other words, if you are a woman you don't want your arms to bulge or become the size of your thigh, and if you are a guy you want to look muscular, but more like the hero than the villain. Well whether you are a man or a woman you still want a flat stomach and you still want to look lean so going to the gym is pretty much non-negotiable. It doesn't just give you aesthetic benefits but even works at building a stronger bone density; that's one benefit you surely want because good bone density helps you anti-age and look 25 at 40. Weight training not only makes your body a better fat burning machine but as you will learn in Chapters 2 and 3, it has been proved to be the best inhibitor of lifestyle disorders, especially diabetes.

Ok, you don't care too much for technicalities and all this density-vensity, but what you do know is that you want to look lean. All right, you will have to work the big daddies then: the legs, back, chest, shoulders. That's when the arms stay in their aukaad, looking exactly the size they ought to, not overpowering your entire appearance with the bulge between shoulders and the elbow competing with your paunch (wicked smile). By the way, stand sideways facing the mirror, the middle of your arm should be bigger than your stomach and smaller than your thigh. That's going to be possible only when you learn to structure your strength training routine in the gym. Till that time, it's gonna be bye-bye arms — arms that continue to move even after the object you said bye to is far from your sight.

Just do 100 suryanamaskars!

Woo ho! Another ortho smiled in a brightly-lit 5-star hospital and kissed his orthoscope. 'Come on! But suryanamaskar is an ancient science and it works the whole spine, stimulating every single chakra in the body and leads to purification of the system … blah blah.' Hold it right there. Stop this bakwas! There isn't one rishi, muni, acharya, text that claims one asana or sequence brings about all of these or even one of the benefits. And even if it does, it does it with a whole lot of '*', that means, conditions apply. Just some of these conditions are that your achar, vichar, ahar — that's conduct, thought and diet — are in tune or at least aligned with the principles of yoga. For example, if you are thinking, 'I really shouldn't be eating this pastry, I just had one yesterday', then in your conduct you can't be standing at the counter paying for it and then in your diet you shouldn't be eating it. Get it?

Fat chance that you will get it and slim chance that you will have a lean waist. Also, let's face it, you are doing this whole 'ancient science' business only because you want to lose weight and that all of those 'benefits' and 'chakras' you rattled off about don't matter more than that number on the weighing scale or fitting into skinny jeans. Here's the truth: the fact that you are putting your body (a very important entity and something worth nurturing and looking after, according to the ancient yogic science) through the rigmarole of 100 suryanamaskars a day only means that you are messing up the technique, the sequence, the balance between your left and right sides and simply focusing on 'sweating it out' or 'burning calories', stuff that the ancient science didn't even bother mentioning and doesn't stand for.

Yes, suryanamaskar does offer benefits from chakra purification to nirvana and everything in between, but when you are not precise, in fact perfect, in your practice of the postures, the ill-effects of doing them wrong are just as enormous. For every celebrity you 'know' who does 100 suryanamaskars, you really KNOW a Sarita who pulled her knee ligament, a Bhushan who injured his back, Anuja who developed scapula tendonitis, and forget all of them, you yourself feel far from thin. Mostly you feel bloated, aggressive, get headaches post noon and have started needing more than your two cups of coffee. Wake up sweetie, you are doing something very wrong here.

So should you never do 100 suryanamaskars? Of course you can! There's a charity called Yoga Aid Challenge through which, from Times Square in New York, to the Darling Harbour in Sydney, right to the banks of the Ganga in Rishikesh, large groups of yoga practitioners meet and perform 108 suryanamaskars to raise money for their favourite cause. But then that's the thing: it's a BIG deal, you perform 108 suryanamaskars as a challenge, you create media attention around it, you spread the word and you spend the rest of the year practising your asanas, sequence, etc. diligently. It's like running a marathon. You do it once in a while, after adequate practice, where you run much less than the 42 km on a daily basis. No prizes for guessing what happens when you run 42 km every day.

So what's a good number to start with? You can start with one, which actually means two, since one on each side — right and left — is counted as one round. Train under a teacher who doesn't push you to achieve a 'number' but pushes you to get your posture right in each of the asanas and teaches you how to breathe through the sequence. Then there's a chance that you may get a fleeting glimpse of all the benefits of the ancient science, and yes, weight loss follows too. God! You really are stuck on your weight, aren't you?

Sweating melts the fat

Wait! Say that again? My li'l baby, didn't you go to school where they taught you that fat (or oil) and water don't mix? So how exactly did this miracle happen in your body, where fat dissolved itself in water that comes out of your pores?

All right, you say, if not fat then let 'toxins' dissolve and come out of our pores mixed in sweat? Ok listen, let's get the basics right. Sweating is a process that takes place in the body as a means of thermoregulation. Bolega toh, when your core body temperature gets heated or goes higher than normal, then as a means of 'cooling off', the body sweats, wherein it loses its water, electrolytes and some minerals too. **Sweat too much and you won't get less fat or more pure or detoxed, but plain dehydrated**. Dehydrate beyond point of repair and you could go straight to hell (for being so foolish about the concept of sweating).

This myth of 'sweating leads to detox or fat loss' is planted deep in our psyche. Now here's what happens: when you work out, the core body temperature does get raised and to keep the body temperature at its optimum, the body will sweat. The fact that the process of sweating exists means that the body's wisdom realizes that for optimum performance, the body temperature should be optimum, not low (to involuntarily shiver) and not too high (to involuntarily sweat). You will notice this in day-to-day life: you don't feel up to things if it's too hot or too cold.

Now exercising in steam rooms or heated environments or without air-conditioning beats the very purpose of exercise. If you are going to spend your time exercising, you would want to optimize or get the best out of your body. Instead you are spending more energy or calories thermo-regulating and not as much in muscle fibre recruitment or performance. So more calories are spent in just ensuring that the vital functions can continue, and that's a waste.

As you read through the book and understand exercise science and its application to your workout, you will, hopefully, be the next myth-buster of your gym / yoga class / running group. Some of the other myths that will be covered in the chapters ahead are:

- Walking is the best exercise
- More time in gym = better body
- Machine-free weight training is better for fat-burning
- Cardio on an empty stomach, or coffee before cardio
- Mixing strength training with cardio
- Marathon training is all about running
- Pranayama, breathing, meditation is yoga
- Doing yoga for specific body parts or with diet restrictions

Chapter 2

Exercise Science — What Happens Behind the Scenes

Not just wholesome meals, you need wholesome workouts too.

The primary goal of exercise is that it brings about muscular contraction. It may seem really superficial and small compared to the complex organism that the human body is, but it is anything but shallow. It has a profound effect on our health, wellbeing and fitness at all levels — physical, mental, emotional and even spiritual. The heart, for example, goes through major adaptations based on the kind of training or exercise program that you subject your body to. Latest research and evidence in real life points conclusively towards the fact that sitting, or plain inactivity, characterized by lack of muscular contraction, is an independent risk factor to developing lifestyle diseases like obesity, diabetes, heart disease, disc prolapse, hernia, blood pressure, arthritis, cancer and everything in between. **Sitting is the new smoking**. Just like smoking was and remains an independent risk factor to obesity, heart disease, cancer and everything in between, so is sitting. Independent risk factor means that, irrespective of 'but I eat home-cooked only', 'work out almost all days ya', 'always sleep at a certain time', 'love my job' and 'don't get stressed easily', if you spend a considerable amount of time sitting / inactive, then you are screwed.

Physical activity

Of course this book is about exercise (I haven't forgotten that), but before we get to that, you must know that lack of physical activity (PA) and the risk that it brings will not be magically washed away by an hour in the gym / park, etc. Exercising doesn't have the effect of Ganga nahaliya so everything maaf. What you do for 23 hours of your day will always have a greater bearing than what you do for 1 hour in the day. Having said that, exercise remains of paramount importance to human life, allowing you to make the most of the remaining 23 hours of the day (and hence this book).

Now, before you start cribbing about how you don't have that 1 hour and how if you had that 1 hour, I wouldn't be making royalty on this book, etc., let me tell you another interesting fact about exercise. **It takes as little as 150 minutes of exercise per week** to improve blood glucose tolerance, reduce body fat and the risk to all possible lifestyle diseases that come with obesity. Through the next few chapters, you will learn how to plan those 150 minutes a week of exercise for yourself, and why it's not as simple as just going for a walk.

Coming back to the topic, an increase in PA for us, as in, Indians living in India, is not all that simple. We mistake inactivity as a necessary expression of our wealth or status in society. The memsahibs who carry LVs don't even have to open the door of their own car to sit in the passenger seat. The big sahib won't rinse his own chai cup because he is either too educated, too rich or too high up in the hierarchy. The less we move, the better it makes us. Much more worthy of respect, power and clout. Really? All that it makes us is people who need to manage their diabetes, BP, thyroid, etc. for 35 years and longer. It turns us into a lazy population and makes lethargy and inactivity aspirational, much like that designer bag or that sea-facing bungalow.

Don't blame your genes

We then take to blaming our genes. 'I am genetically prone to obesity, diabetes, etc.' Somehow we never bother 'blaming' our genes for the marks we earned in school, for our IQ, for the promotion you got last week. No, no — all that is your ability and hard work. Well, obesity is exactly the lack of hard work, or maybe the perverted hard work you put into not moving your body or moving it as little as possible. There are people who won't get out of their office chair till the lift has been called and is waiting for them, the car is in the porch parked as close to the exit door as possible and the driver is holding the door open for you. Wow! You sure made it large — and by 'it' I mean your stomach and your expenditure on pharmaceutical drugs, one to let you sleep in the night, the other to wake you up in the morning, others to keep the BP and blood sugar down, and thyroid up. Well done!

Most gene studies have focused on body weight and not on body composition, and such constrained studies don't paint the right picture. In fact, most gene studies only teach the researchers how to design the next gene study better. Identical twins with the same set of genes but different levels of physical activities have dramatically different body weight and risks to diseases. So forget genes — good or bad, you can't change them; for now, just take this new medicine, it's called activity. Just move more and sit less.

Time and again, it has been proved that scientific information doesn't bring about a change in behaviour. Behaviour, after all, is not rocket science; it's not as simple ;). Ok, I heard this line at a fitness conference: if you like it and maro it, know that it's not mine, it's by a guy from Sao Paulo — they seem to say and do all the right things there. Anyway, change in exercise and PA behaviour or attitude cannot be brought about by scientific evidence but by a change of heart. And like all good things, it starts at home. So be a man and clean up the kitchen every Sunday, work side-by-side with your sister, mother, wife and take an active part in sharing household responsibilities on a daily basis, including cooking, cleaning, washing, ironing, etc. Given the fact that most of us have house help, this is not going to amount to a lot of work, but it will result in two main things: 1. Allow you to accumulate PA and all its associated benefits (in addition to envious glances from neighbours and endless compliments on being a cool guy), and 2. It gives the women in the household a chance to be in a nurturing environment where there is respect and scope for them to pursue their fitness too.

Anyway man or woman, home or office, it's important to stay physically active and not confuse it with exercise. They are vastly different but equally important, and doing one doesn't make up for not doing the other. Ghar ki safaee, kitchen ke kaam, jhadoo-poncha don't make up for pushing weights in the gym, or learning to lift the waist in trikonasana, or doing a sprint interval in the sand. It's like this, **PA makes us fit enough to age and exercise reverses ageing**. Believe it or not, most of us are so weak in our bones, so poor with our memory, so stiff in our backs and so messed up with our blood sugars that we are not even fit enough to age. Some of us are barely in our mid-20s and already have a disc-prolapse; some of us in our 30s have trouble keeping our cholesterol in check; not even 45, and heart is already enlarged and BP pills are a part of the daily diet. See, we are all going to live long enough thanks to 'drugs and technology', but with that increased lifespan, are we only going to occupy hospital beds or pay our hard-earned money to pharma companies?

But it's not so grim, the body changes the minute you change your mind and embrace PA and exercise as a way of life. For example, **in as little as 48 hours post exercise, there's improvement in insulin sensitivity**. Now show me a drug that can do that in as little time and with no side effects other than the feeling of wellbeing.

Film-star thin

You are never gonna look like SRK, Saif, Salman — no, not because you are not a Khan, but because you don't belong to the filmi profession. Films, I think, are the only place where the more successful you get, the more physically active you have to be on your sets. You are in almost every frame of the movie, you are called all the time on the set so you walk from your van to the shot, you spend a lot of time standing around before your shot, till they fix the lighting, move the camera, check for sound, etc. Your work entails standing, walking, moving, dancing, fighting, emoting and very little sitting. Along with that, given the fact that you are an actor, you have naturally high kinaesthetic intelligence and you look forward to exercise on most days. End result: you look leaner, fitter, younger than most people of your age.

Acting is a physical job and that's exactly why out-of-work actors get fat. No acting, no fat-burning.

Also, it is helpful to remember that most of these guys have been working and working out for years. I would see Saif weight train even when I was consulting at The Club (found him charming even then, and since then my love for him has only grown), and that was sometime in 2001; it's 2013 now. What someone looks like after 12 years of consistent training, you are not going to achieve in 12 days.

The best exercise

I am often asked, 'But according to you, what is the best exercise?' **Very simply, the best exercise is the one that gets done on a regular basis**. If you are a lover of the breaststroke in an Olympic-size pool, then that's the best exercise for you. If you love the treadmill, then it's the treadmill for you. If squatting under a bar double your body weight does it for you, then it's weight training for you, and if your head won't function without the sirsasana / sarvangasana cycle, then it's yoga for you. It's like asking me who is the best person for you to marry, I won't know that. But anyone you love and who holds your interest is a good bet; same goes for exercise.

However, **it's one thing for something to qualify as the best exercise but quite another for you to be the best at it.** It's like this, and we have all seen this way too often in life — you look and look and finally you find your dream man / woman, who hooks your interest, gives you a sense of purpose and accomplishment and makes life worth living. You want to spend all your time waking, sleeping, dreaming with this person. Your friends complain that you don't meet them that often, your cousin is upset that you won't return her calls, you are distracted at work and the boss is going crazy but you couldn't care less. You have found what you were looking for, you have found happiness! But in less than two months you are not quite sure if this is 'happiness'; the man / woman of your dreams is giving you nightmares, you want to meet your cousin / friend and vent, but you have pushed them so far away that you feel alone in this painful situation. You find yourself keeping away from this person, avoiding calls, being distracted at dinner, etc., and feel that ending this relationship is the only solution. You probably do end it too, only to go into a repeat mode with another person; script, drama and ending, intact.

To live with that love forever means that you keep your interest in work, friends and cousins alive and active. After all, your dream man / woman doesn't crack up at your jokes like your cousin does, doesn't find the hairdresser super-sexy like you and your friend do, and doesn't pay you like your boss does. So the only way to stay in love is to look after every other aspect of one's life and relationships. Now just replace 'person' with running / tennis / yoga / gymming / Zumba / dancing, your love or choice of exercise and you will see what I am talking about. To stay with your 'best' exercise forever, you have to look after every fitness parameter. Every exercise is limited in its design and cannot look after the different components of fitness — endurance, strength, flexibility and cardio-respiratory — equally well. Invariably, it over-trains one of the components and under-trains the other. For example, running will improve stamina and endurance but does nothing to build strength or flexibility. Lack of strength and flexibility will come in the way of your running. Eventually a shin split may keep you off running for weeks and lead you to lose out on stamina too. Or you are really good at tennis, but your forehand may lose its power because of stiffness in your Achilles tendon, which prevents you from shifting your weight behind that racquet.

A well-rounded exercise plan employs all the energy systems in our body. As we will learn shortly, the human body consists of three different energy systems or types of metabolism, but broadly they are classified as the aerobic and the anaerobic systems. Depending on the task at hand, your body chooses which energy system should be employed. One of the main reasons why most people feel burnt out or risk an injury with their best exercise is because they don't maintain a balance between the different energy systems. They build one at the cost of the other.

Cardio over 'others'?

An extension of the 'best exercise' question is, 'But isn't cardio the best exercise?' It is definitely the most recommended exercise by dieticians, physicians, nephrologists, cardiologists and the like who have over-simplified the effects and benefits of an endurance / cardio program. On the other hand, **the benefits of an anaerobic program are not well known** outside the exercise science and physiology world, and this leads to it not just being 'not recommended', but also actively discouraged by health professionals with a 'marne ka hai kya' or 'back tod ne ka hai?' I mean, they take the Kaikayee approach from *Ramayana*: 'Bharat ko raaj, Ram ko vanvaas.' Bharat ko raaj tak theek hai, why Ram ko vanvaas? Declaring and promoting 'walking' as the best exercise is ok and a forgivable indulgence, laughable even, but the active discouragement, clicking of the tongue, frowning of the forehead and disapproving shake of the head for activities like weight training, sprinting, forward-bending, inversions come out of the bias and fear of the unknown rather than any real threat or danger to your health.

By learning about the energy systems explained ahead in the chapter, you will understand that training the anaerobic pathways offers not just benefits to your strength and looks but also to your heart and lungs. You will also learn how some of the training adaptations to both aerobic and anaerobic programs will dramatically improve your heart health and how a basic knowhow of exercise can rid you from this 'I am a blood report' mentality.

Dil ki baat

Now if you really want to improve the condition of your heart, lower your blood pressure, improve blood circulation, lose body fat, improve the health of your kidney, lungs, whatever your personal goal is, you need to train both the aerobic and the anaerobic pathways. It's the anaerobic pathways that are employed when you perform 'hard' activities like sprints, trekking uphill, weight training, learning to go up in sirsasana, etc., and the heart responds by making the adaptations mentioned above. But before that, a little about the heart.

So the heart sits a little leftish of your chest cavity, is the size of your fist, and bears the responsibility of receiving and pumping blood to the entire body, all the way from your brain to your little toe. It can be roughly divided into four distinct chambers, each one performing a unique task. The upper two chambers are called auricles and the lower chambers are called ventricles; and these are then subdivided as right auricle, right ventricle and left auricle and left ventricle.

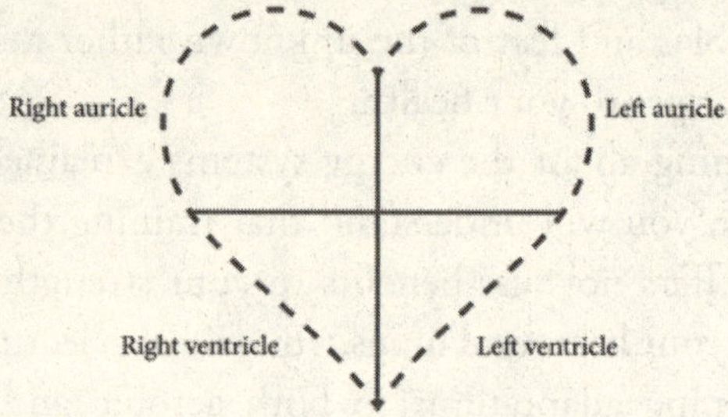

The left ventricle is the lower, left chamber of the heart and is the one currently of interest to us. This is the chamber that pumps oxygenated blood to the body. The changes that this chamber goes through in response to exercise are what the doctors describe as 'good for the heart', and exercise physiologists as 'hypertrophy'. Simply put, this means the increase in size and strength of the heart muscle.

As a response to the endurance or aerobic or cardio programs, the left ventricle will go through an increase in size and become bigger than what it was. **But, and this is crucial, it's with non-endurance or anaerobic training (gymming, sprinting, etc.) that the left ventricle will also develop a thicker wall, with a larger and more efficient capillary network, leading to an increase in strength as well.** For improvements in heart health, both training adaptations, that of a larger ventricular cavity and strength of the wall, are essential. Only then will there be a real decrease in blood lipid profile, BP, blood sugar, etc. Till that time you will continue needing that goli. Doing one, in fact overdoing one, like going for a walk every day and never sprinting or strength training, is a half-hearted attempt to improve heart health.

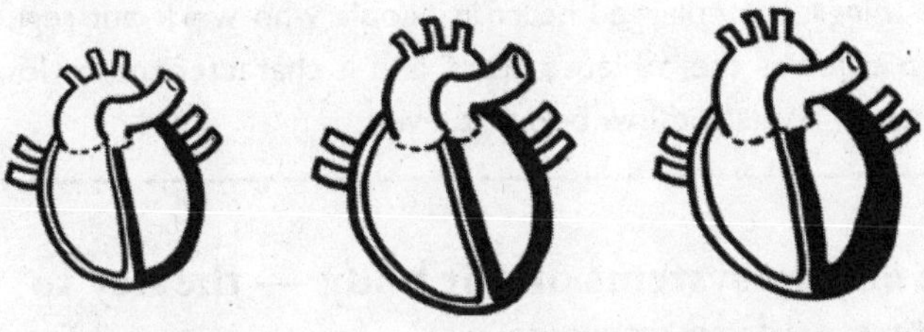

Untrained heart | Trained heart – aerobic only – increase in size | Trained heart – aerobic and anaerobic – increase in size and thickness of LV

It's also true that people who don't exercise have both, a small and weak wall in the left ventricle (LV). Chalo, LV gets a new meaning altogether now ☺. Hope you get the point that all energy systems must be utilized to get benefits out of your exercise program, no more half-hearted attempts people. Below is a further explanation of these energy systems and how they differ from each other, and just like the heart, their effect on other organs and systems of your body is also 'alag che'.

Technical note — Enlarged heart / Athlete's paradox

Enlarged heart is a common heart ailment, an adaptation that the kind heart goes through in response to hypertension or high blood pressure. This enlarged heart is often seen in sedentary individuals, with little or no exercise and high body weight and is identified as a serious risk to the heart. Now athletic training or even recreational exercise can bring about the exact same adaptation — enlarged heart. The difference is that, in people who work out, the heart enlarges because it gets bigger in size, strength and vascularity, and in sedentary folk it enlarges to make up for the lack of the exact same things. The enlarged heart in people who work out regularly is also called as the 'athlete's heart' and is characterized by low or normal BP levels and low body fat levels.

The energy systems of our body — the key to understanding exercise

Even before you plan your workout, you need to understand the energy systems that the body employs to help you perform the exercise. I am going to keep this as simple as I can, but it's of paramount importance that you take time to understand it. In fact, let me put it this way, one of the reasons why people come to me for advice on exercise and nutrition is exactly because I understand the basics of exercise physiology (and cross my heart, I am still learning, and God knows I have a lot more to learn). It's this understanding that will put you in a unique position of advantage where you will learn how much and what type of exercise you should do to optimize fat-burning. Essentially it will teach you how to spend less time exercising and more time collecting compliments.

So, broadly, your body produces energy in three different ways to carry out any task / activity / exercise you undertake. **The intensity of your activity will decide which energy system will dominate, but at any given time all three will be in use.** Think of them as production, marketing and sales

— all three work at all times, but depending on the task, one of them will work more than the other.

Here is what your energy systems are called:

<table>
<tr><td>1. Aerobic system</td><td></td></tr>
<tr><td>2. Glycogen-Lactic acid system</td><td rowspan="2">} Anaerobic systems</td></tr>
<tr><td>3. ATP-CP system</td></tr>
</table>

The aerobic system, well, follows the aerobic pathway, and by that it means that muscles get to use oxygen. This pathway was developed to carry out tasks that go on for a long time, for example to equip you with the stamina to walk from one village to another or from your home to school or at least from the car park to the movie theatre ☺, or in sports like long-distance running, etc. So this system can help you carry out tasks that are not high in intensity but high in volume. If you are sitting or even lying down (sit up if you are) while reading this book, you are using the aerobic pathway.

The ATP-CP and glycogen-lactic acid system follow the anaerobic pathway, which means that they function in the absence of oxygen. Absence of oxygen doesn't mean there is no oxygen available, it only means that the task was completed so fast, oxygen couldn't reach the working muscle group. Working without oxygen means that the muscles will be able to work for a very short duration of time because there is only so much you can sustain in the absence of oxygen. Since they last for a very short period of time, obviously they can carry out really high-intensity tasks.

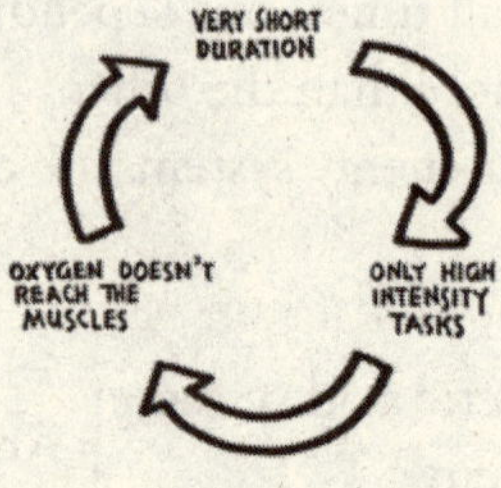

In fact, one of the reasons why the human body created this metabolic pathway or energy system is because there are a whole lot of high-intensity activities that we need to carry out in a very short duration. For example, a tight slap that you may need to strike on the bus because the molester just squeezed your glutes, or the dash that you have to make for the remote or lose control to your irritating sibling and be forced to watch F1 again ☺, or in sports like sprinting and jumping.

This is a rather simplified version of these metabolic pathways. Needless to say, there are a whole lot of different enzymes, fuel substrates, electron transfer systems, muscle fibre types, genetics, training and environment factors, etc. involved, most of which is beyond the scope of this book (oh God! I feel so hi-funda saying that ;)). So for now we are going to focus on understanding the two most crucial ones: fuel and muscle type. We need to understand these two to gain a better understanding of these pathways and, more importantly, to make an intelligent choice about exercise. So that hum kam kaam kare aur zyada patle lage ;). Smartass trainers call this **train smart and not hard, know which energy system to manipulate** and how to bring about maximum fat loss, or shall I say 'results'.

Fuel and muscle type

Now when you say that body toned lagna chahiye, you essentially mean that you need to develop more muscle mass than you currently have. And you say that because, deep down in the deepest reservoir of your brain and heart, you know that muscle is THE only metabolic active tissue in your body. The one entity that revs up your metabolism, burns your fat, makes you look young, attractive, hot and keeps you fertile is muscle.

And this muscle comes in two different types (yeah! welcome to exercise physiology class); they're called the oxidative and the non-oxidative muscle fibres or the red and the white fibres or the slow and fast twitch fibres, or if you want to sound very technical then Type 1 and Type 2 fibres. The Type 2 fibres are further divided as Type 2a and Type 2b fibres. It seems complicated because you never paid so much attention to exercise as a science. It is one nevertheless, and your trainer deserves that fee he / she is asking for. (And for peanuts you get monkeys not trainers.) Anyway this science is easier than the algorithms you cracked (yeah, yeah if I can get it, it's a no-brainer).

The aerobic system employs the Type 1 or slow twitch (ST) muscle fibres that can contract and carry out work for longer periods of time. Since it operates in the presence of oxygen, it can burn carbohydrate, protein and fat as a fuel to derive energy. These have a lot of mitochondria, things which help you oxidize fat and also give it the red appearance. So,

Type 1 / Slow twitch / Red — Low intensity / Long duration aerobic — Carb / Fat / Protein as fuel

The Type 2 or the fast twitch (FT) muscle fibres don't have as much mitochondria so they work when you are using the anaerobic energy system. Since they don't have too much mitochondria or myoglobin (this is the cousin of haemoglobin and found inside the muscle tissue; like Hb, this myoglobin binds to oxygen too, forming O_2-myoglobin), they appear less red or, in fact, white. The glycogen-lactic acid system employs the Type 2a muscle fibres and, as the name suggests, they use carbs in the form of glycogen stored in muscle and liver as fuel. Type 2a are the most versatile muscle fibres and keep the ability to use / generate forces both aerobically and anerobically. The ATP-CP or the alactic acid system employs the Type 2b fibre type and uses the stored and ready-to-use energy molecule Adenosine Triphosphate (ATP) to produce really quick energy in a short span of time. So,

Type 2 / Fast twitch / White — High intensity / Short duration — Glycogen / ATP as fuel

---

Technical note – Type of fuel

There are basically three types of fuels or sources of energy that the body uses:

1. ATP-CP

ATP (Adenosine Triphosphate) is a readily available and stored molecule in our muscles. It consists of an adenosine component and 3 'high energy' phosphate groups and can be represented as below::

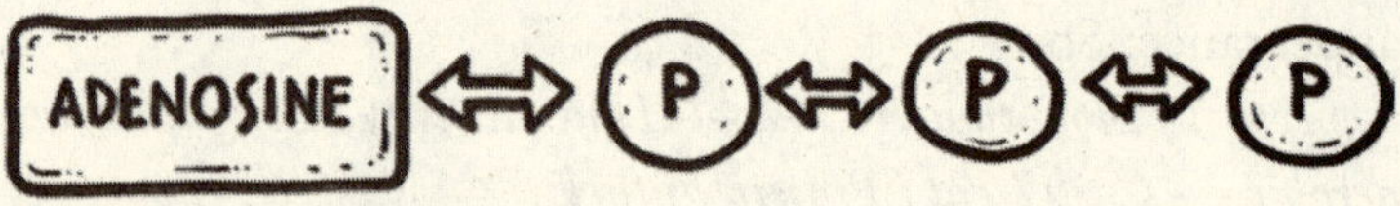

When the muscles need energy, they break down one of the phosphate bonds, resulting in 1 ADP molecule, a free phosphate and significant amount of energy.

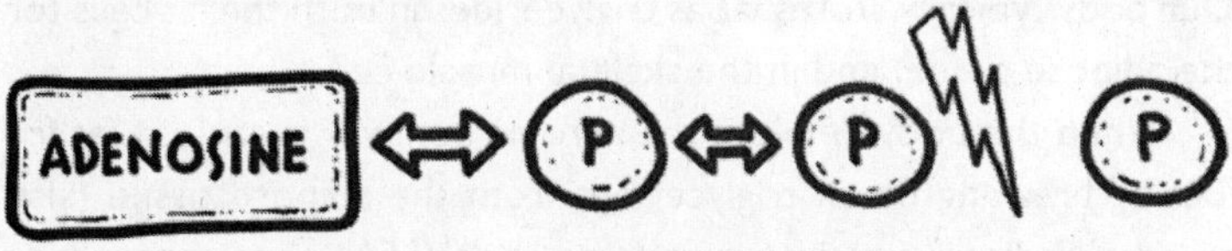

Another chemical that provides stored energy is Creatine Phosphate (CP). However, the cells can't use CP directly, but instead use it for conversion of ADP to ATP. Like ATP, CP is also in short supply and needs to be constantly resynthesized.

The ATP-CP cycle is not dependent on the presence of oxygen and is therefore extremely important for anaerobic type of activities. Because it is readily available in the muscles for use, the body relies on this when it has to perform any task quickly, in a short duration of time.

2. Carbs

Carbs from food are broken down into glucose, which is transported through blood and stored in the muscles and liver as glycogen (cluster of glucose molecules).

In the absence of oxygen (anaerobic metabolism), 1 glucose molecule at a time from glycogen is broken down into an intermediate product called pyruvic and then to lactic acid, and the energy produced during this reaction generates ATP (2 molecules of ATP for every glucose molecule).

In the presence of oxygen (aerobic metabolism), the pyruvic acid doesn't get converted to lactic acid; instead, after a series of reactions, to carbon dioxide and water plus 36 molecules of ATP.

So aerobically more energy (ATP) can be produced per molecule of glucose as compared to anaerobic. Also, aerobically there are fewer exercise by-products than anaerobic (which produces the muscle-fatiguing lactic acid).

3. Fats

Our body typically stores fat as triglycerides in both the fat cells (or the adipose tissue) and in the skeletal muscle cell.

When the body employs the aerobic pathway it can use fat for fuel by breaking down triglycerides from the adipose tissue (also called as adipocytes) into free fatty acids (FFA) and transporting it via the blood to the working muscle tissue where they are converted to ATP. One FFA produces 147 ATP molecules.

Aerobically, when fat is broken down it produces more energy (147 ATP) as compared to carbs (36 ATP per glucose molecule).

Anaerobically, fat cannot be used as a fuel but when performing anaerobic activity with intervening rest periods, the FFA from blood play a minor role as energy source.

4. Proteins

Technically, the body can use protein as a source of fuel too (aerobically). However, it is used as a fuel only in extreme conditions and mostly used for its main purpose — that of building and repairing body tissue. It has been estimated that not more than 5-10% of the body's total energy comes from protein.

Summary

So what you need to remember is that, for anaerobic pathway, pre-stored ATP and glycogen are the only sources of fuel. For the aerobic pathway, all three — carbs, fats and proteins — can be used as fuel. Although aerobically fat appears to be the most important source of fuel, the fact that carbs are more efficient (need fewer oxygen molecules for oxidation) makes them more important as the starting fuel, with fat taking over later. That's exactly why it is always said that fat is burned on the carbohydrate flame ☺.

The miracle of after-burn

You all must be like, 'Ya, thanks for all the gyaan and thanks for making exercise more complicated than it already was! But can I please know what will burn maximum calories for me — aerobic or anaerobic, that was the whole point of buying this book, to lose fat, lose weight and fit into tighter clothes.'

Ok, two things — a) we are getting to that shortly and b) it is not so straightforward, but it's not complicated either. Remember our deal? If I can get it, so can you ☺.

You burn calories as a result of any activity. But it's not all that easy to calculate EEE (Exercise Energy Expenditure), a technical and more complete term for calories burnt. Yes, don't let the treadmill display fool you into believing that you actually burned 500kcals or get swayed by the random calculations like consuming 500kcals less per day will lead to weight loss.

Calculating energy expenditure cannot be reduced to a mathematical formula; there are many factors that influence your energy expenditure — more relevant to our topic, energy expenditure during exercise. Some of these are age, sex, body composition, pre-workout meal, meal history through the week, basically it's all quite overwhelming and the research is still in progress. Which means that exercise physiologists, people with sharp brains, sharper equipment and research budgets to match are not quite sure how many calories you have actually burned. Your treadmill, the Sexy Sam in your gym or your dietician aunty, on the other hand, seem much more certain about it. So you decide who is better informed about the whole process.

But what we do know is that: a) Exercise Energy Expenditure (EEE) is a combination of calories burned during exercise and calories burned after or due to exercise. And b) Calories burned are directly proportional to oxygen consumed (this is how calories burned is measured in labs).

So the two parts of EEE are:

1. Calories burned during exercise

During aerobic activity – Oxygen consumption increases and therefore calories are burned. Oxygen uptake is also proportional to the heat expenditure during exercise. This is also why you sweat (expend heat) much more during aerobic type of activities like a long run or a dance class.

And during anaerobic activity – Oxygen consumption is less and therefore less calories are burned.

2. Calories burned post exercise

For aerobic activity – Hardly any extra oxygen is consumed above what is needed at rest.

And for anaerobic activity – Post exercise, a lot more oxygen is needed to restore the body to its resting state (breathing, circulation, digestion, hormones, etc.), and to adapt to the exercise by recovering and repairing from the microscopic tissue damage (anabolism). This is called **oxygen debt** (or oxygen debit these days) — also known as EPOC (Excess Post-exercise Oxygen Consumption) — or a more popular term, **after-burn.**

This can be represented as below:

Type of exercise	Calories burned	
	During exercise	After exercise / Due to exercise
Aerobic	More	Very little
Anaerobic	Less	**A whole lot more due to after-burn**

So oxygen debt, or after-burn, or the extra oxygen required post exercise as compared to oxygen required at rest, is the crucial factor here. And it is further divided into two parts

a) Alactic acid debt: Amount of oxygen required to replenish the ATP–CP stores in the muscles. This is carried out aerobically and happens quickly in about three to four minutes of stopping exercise. This is called the rapid segment of the oxygen debt.

b) Lactic acid debt: This is linked to the amount of lactic acid that gets produced during exercise and is dependent on intensity, duration and type of exercise. EPOC does the job of removing lactic acid accumulation from the muscles, restoring glycogen stores, bringing body temperature back to resting state, etc. This is the slow segment of the oxygen debt and can take up to 24 to 48 hours based on the intensity of workout. In other words, due to performing anaerobic activity, your body will burn more calories (or even simpler, burn more fat) for as long as 24 to 48 hours post exercise.

Obviously, then, it's not just about 'sweating it out' or 'burning 500 calories'; you have to factor in the after-burn too, which is based on multiple variables. But what we do know is that **after-burn for anaerobic activities is exponentially higher than what it is for aerobic exercise**. Essentially the amount of fat you will burn or how much fat-burning you will achieve and therefore the final effect on your body composition (how thin, actually how lean and young you look) is based on the accumulative effect of after-burn through the week.

Now don't be quick to jump the gun and declare that if fat-burning and looking thin is your goal then it only makes sense to train the anaerobic pathway. You will at all times need to train both the aerobic and the anaerobic pathways, and know that both influence the efficiency of each other, and therefore the fat-burning effects of one another (you will learn how in the next few chapters). ***In short, just like wholesome meals, you need wholesome workouts too.***

Summary of energy systems

Ok, here is the table you can refer to for all that we have discussed on energy systems.

Energy systems	Aerobic	Anaerobic	
		Glycogen-lactic acid system	ATP-CP system
Energy production (ATP)	**Unlimited**	**Limited**	**Very limited**

Energy systems	**Aerobic**	**Anaerobic**	
		Glycogen-lactic acid system	**ATP-CP system**
Fuel used	**Carb, fat, protein (in this order)**	**Carbs (as glycogen)**	**ATP, CP, Glycogen**
Also	Can consume lactic acid	Produces lactic acid and Creatine Phosphate (CP)	Consumes CP
After-burn	**Very little**	**High**	**High**
Muscle fibre type	**Type 1**	**Type 2a**	**Type 2b**
Contraction ability	Slow	Fast	Very fast
Mitochondria density and myoglobin	Very high	Medium	Low
Activity	**Long-term aerobic**	**Long-term anaerobic**	**Short bursts of anaerobic activity**
Duration	Endless / hours together	Lasts for max 1-3 minutes	Less than 30 seconds
Example in sports	Marathon	Middle-distance running, up to 800m	Sprints

Energy systems	**Aerobic**	**Anaerobic**	
		Glycogen-lactic acid system	**ATP-CP system**
Examples of activities more relevant for me	**Cardio or endurance training**	**Interval training, weight-training, sports at competitive level**	**Power training or heavy weight-training, sprint training or jumps**

Now I want you to remember only what I've marked in BOLD, because that is what is relevant to us, to the choices of exercises we make, to the kind of fuel we want to burn, to the way we want to look. The only reason why I put some more info than what is immediately relevant is because these factors are important and lead us to the relevant points.

Table: Performance time and dominant energy systems

Here is a quick reference table which shows the energy system involved in various activities / exercises based on their performance time.

Performance time	**Major energy systems involved**	**Examples**
Less than 30 sec	ATP-CP	Shot put, 100m sprint, Tennis swings

30 – 90 sec	ATP-CP and Lactic acid	400m sprint, 100m swim
90 sec – 3 min	Lactic acid and aerobic	800m run, gymnastics, boxing, wrestling
> 3 mins	Aerobic	Marathon, jogging, long swims

Table: Various sports (competitive) and percentage contribution of energy systems

Sports	ATP-CP	Lactic acid	Aerobic
Basketball	85	15	-
Hockey	60	20	20
Football	90	10	-
Golf swing	95	5	-
Gymnastics	90	10	-
Tennis	70	20	10
Recreational sports Tennis / Squash / Frisbee / Basketball / Badminton / Cricket, etc., when we play in clubs / societies / mohallas, etc.	-	5	95

Energy systems and exercise myths

Ok, let's quickly summarize what we learnt in energy systems above:

1. Different exercises or types of activities use different types of muscle fibres and fuel.
2. All types of muscle fibres must be put to use if you want to look and feel fit.
3. While aerobic exercises can use fat as fuel while exercising (in addition to carbs and proteins), anaerobic activities can burn fat for as long as 48 hours after exercise (called after-burn).

Most injuries, fads and 'experiments' with exercise come out of 'boredom' / overtraining, which in turn can be attributed to bad workout planning, which in turn stems from no understanding of the energy systems of the body. Basically, if you understand energy systems, you can stop yourself doing silly things with your exercise routine.

No understanding of energy systems → Bad workout planning → Fads and injuries

Let's look at some of the common myths once again and understand them from the energy systems perspective.

1. Sweating more for more fat loss

You can now see that sweating is not the same as fat melting, it is only about the heat generated during any type of activity, and aerobic activity produces heat proportional to oxygen consumed. So you are likely to sweat more during aerobic types of activities, but because it comes with little or less after-burn (EPOC) as compared to anaerobic activities, it is going to mean less fat burning.

Creating conditions where you sweat in excess basically reduces your ability to exercise or burn calories at its optimum.

So working out without an AC or with all the windows closed and fan switched off, wearing a hood over your head while running, wearing dark, tight clothes, choosing yoga classes (or any workout) based on which allows you to sweat more, are all practices that need to be abandoned right away because these are counterproductive to not just the body's fat-burning abilities but also to all the fitness parameters.

2. Spot reduction — many reps for one body part

For example, leg lifts to reduce the outer thigh and crunches for a flat stomach.

When you are able to lift anything for 15 reps and more it is in the aerobic zone (Chapter 3). Now the crunch and the leg lift and the doggy and whatever you do, you can do 20, who knows 50, even 200 reps per set. What energy system have you employed? Aerobic! What fuel have you used? Glycogen, fat and protein, and in that order.

So have you burned fat on top of the thigh or stomach? No, you've burned free fatty acids (FFA) from the blood stream, and much more than that, you've burned the glycogen stores. Of course, accompanied by jarring of joints and overuse of the muscle in use. And will there be a surge in the FFA utilization post exercise? No! Because this 'exercise' is not going to give you after-burn.

And what is worth remembering is that the body has an inherent wisdom, a code almost, which decides from what body part the FFA will be mobilized, based on your lifestyle, eating habits and workout intensity. It is no surprise then that people who punish their 'stubborn fat' areas see least reduction in those body parts. That's because of the poor intensity of exercise, no utilization of anaerobic pathway, no after-burn and no essential fat in the diet.

Invariably those who believe that spot reduction is possible are the ones who also avoid ghee and coconut in their diet. More and more 'research' is proving what your grandmom always knew — coconut leads to a slimmer waist and ghee will ensure mobilization of fats from 'stubborn' areas, basically give you a nice proportionate figure. So other than these two miracles, there is no 'miracle' exercise / procedure / tuck for those stubborn spots.

3. Working out twice a day — morning and evening — to burn more calories

So what have we learned about calorie burning? Exercise Energy Expenditure is not just about calories burned during exercise but after as well, till the body is restored to its resting state, where hormones, gas exchange, digestion, circulation, breathing, every parameter returns to normal. Ok, so you do know this and you also understand that the body is still recovering or in EPOC post anaerobic workout, but then why not twice a day cardio, it doesn't have too much EPOC? Here's why:

If you have done your cardio workout well, then you still have some glycogen replenishment to do before the next workout. But fuel aspect apart, factors like recovery of the nerve fibres, tendons, ligaments, joints, bones and even the brain are important. After all, what we want is a toned body, not a broken one. So spare a thought not just for the fuel and therefore the bio-energetic pathways but also for the other bio-mechanical pathways that workouts employ. It's important to be consistent, not stupid with exercise.

4. Dieting and walking

All too often in your zest to lose weight, you visit your dietician and she promptly puts you on a low-calorie, low-carb, low-fat diet. Your doctor also looks down upon anaerobic programs or 'tough' yoga classes and tells you to simply take a walk. Walk, just walk every day for an hour, says the holistic health guru too. Or if it's one of those 'famous' ones, then 'one hour in the morning and one hour in the evening.'

Now before we look at what happens physiologically, let's make time for some bitching. Bitching, btw, is good for the heart, light on the stomach and good for the fat-burning processes too! Boss, if you've got two bloody hours to walk morning and evening you deserve to get and stay fat. Saala! Dharati pe bojh! Why don't you make yourself more useful? Have you forgotten your hobbies? Your dreams? Isn't there something you want to learn? Photography? Tabla? Astronomy? Molecular chemistry? How about cleaning the windows? Visiting your aunt in Pune? Volunteering for the PTA? Or finishing that application for the online designing course from NYU? Or doing that part-time MBA? Sadly, this affects more women than men. You tell a man to walk for two hours daily to lose weight, chances are he will pass. He has work to do. But women? They have started imagining that they are sitting free. While most of their dreams, aspirations, hobbies rot. Bitching ends.

Speaking purely in terms of exercise physiology, you are better off keeping your brain alert, active and involved in skills and activities it wants to learn, improve on and master. The reason being, the human brain is the most metabolically active tissue in the human body per unit square area. So really, even if it's difficult, make time to learn, pursue and practise your hobby / chase your dream. As you invest time in learning the new activity or getting better at an old skill, the brain responds by increasing the number of neurons and mitochondria, so it can actually help you burn more calories too.

Use your brain

Availability of carbohydrates to the brain affects your ability to produce ATP, the metabolic capsule, or the instant source of energy that muscles use to bring about contraction and carry on with exercise. **On a low-carb diet, when you keep walking for hours as a means of losing weight, you risk much more than wasting time**. The brain experiences fatigue because of the lack of glucose availability, leading to headaches (short-term) and loss of memory, faster ageing (long-term), and reduces your body's ability to produce ATP needed for exercise. Though with walking you are in the aerobic zone and technically capable of burning carbs, fat and protein to carry on with exercise, in the absence of adequate dietary supply of carbs, fat and calories, this metabolic priority system takes a beating.

Ideally, not more than 10% of energy should come from burning protein, but in the case of low-carb, low-fat and low-calorie diets, much more than 10% of energy contribution comes from the breaking down of protein. Amino acids, the building blocks of protein, are picked up from existing muscle stores and sacrificed for the act of energy production which will finally produce ATP, allowing muscles to contract and continue with exercise

— that one-hour walk. This loss of muscle tissue leads to a detrimental effect on the bone tissue too and promotes premature ageing in the body. **The whole point of exercise is to promote build-up of muscle and bone tissue and loss of fat mass.** But a low-carb, low-fat diet causes the exact opposite and leads to weight loss at the cost of strength, balance, flexibility, and endurance, as well as to endless fatigue. It's time we understand that exercise can't be over-simplified to 'just go for a walk', though walking is and should remain an all-important means of locomotion / activity. Nothing in exercise physiology goes in favour of walking over other forms of exercise.

The application of the basics of exercise science is important to building a good exercise program and therefore good health and fitness levels. Health and fitness have no bearing on body weight (only to what is contributing to body weight, your body composition), and body weight has no bearing on an individual's health, fitness and wellbeing. When you are sick, hospitalized or terminally ill, you may lose lots of body weight, but it is silly even to think that the weight loss may automatically make you healthier, feel better, lead to better responses from your heart, liver, kidney, etc. Essentially, body weight is a useless thing to lose. There is absolutely no correlation whatsoever between body composition and body weight. Any diet (or spa wellness program or health farm) that doesn't promote exercise and uses only 'diet control' and 'walks' to help you lose weight will not bring down your risk factors to lifestyle diseases.

Technical note — Brain and exercise

As we reach the age of 30, we actually see a drop in our neurons and the nerve tissue in the brain, and the size of our hippocampus, the centre of learning and memory in the brain, decreases. But that's exactly where exercise comes to the rescue. The stress that regular exercises places on our cells leads to an increase in the BDNF (Brain Derived Neurotrophic Factor) gene which leads to a surge in BDNF proteins and promotes neurogenesis — the birth of new neurons. Along with that, it keeps our existing neurons alive and kicking and improves the efficiency of our learning and memory. So you will be quicker at picking up new activities and learning your way around new gadgets, and not stare at people's faces and struggle with names.

The BDNF is also responsible for the analgesic or the pain-blocking effect that exercise brings about. Moreover, BDNF also increases the levels of dopamine (a neurotransmitter) and goes a long way in not just making us 'feel good' or euphoric post exercise, but also in preventing Alzheimer's and Parkinson's. The feel-good and pain-blocking effects that exercise gives can be compared to that of marijuana, but because exercise gratification is delayed (you feel good only post 30 minutes or so), it doesn't get as addictive. In our culture of instant gratification, we seem to be losing out on the patience to 'endure' exercise for 30 minutes before the euphoria sets in, but then some things in life are worth waiting for. World over exercise is now gaining significance as a brain activity and not just a physical activity.

Note – most studies have used aerobic exercise to study the brain's response, but the anaerobic pathway leads to the same feel-good effects and euphoria too.

Some important concepts of exercise science

In addition to understanding the energy systems, there are some other important aspects of exercise science that will enable us to plan and optimize our workout and ensure that there is progress, and not injuries and stagnation.

1. The Borg scale

Of course for us laymen, it becomes difficult to tell whether we are using the aerobic or the anaerobic pathway to produce muscle contraction, and that's exactly where the Borg scale comes in use. Developed by Gunnar Borg, this scale allows you to gauge the pathway or the bioenergetics system employed without using expensive equipment, like heart rate monitors, etc. The Borg scale is also referred to as the Rate of Perceived Exertion (RPE), which accounts for the fact that it is not the task or exercise at hand but your body's response to it that makes it hard, easy or moderate. It also allows for keeping exercise more real, as the task that you rate today at 8 (let's say cycling up Pali Hill) will become 6 after consistent practise over a couple of months. Alternatively, when the body has not recovered from the previous day's workout or a late-night party, a task that usually feels like a 6 may go to an 8. The Borg or RPE scale then serves the dual purpose of:

a) Letting you gauge the bioenergetics and therefore the EPOC and
b) Preventing over-exercising / overtraining and injuries. Obviously when a task of 6 goes to 8, it means you are risking injury, and when a task of 8 falls to 6, it means you have improved and can add more challenges to your exercise. Well done!

Traditionally, it is rated as 0-20, but for all practical purposes, a scale of 0-10 is used.

Rating Rate of Perceived Exertion RPE / Borg scale		
1 2 3 4	Very, very light Fairly light	Sitting or lying down / Little or no effort Walking around / light PA
5 6 7 8	Comfortably uncomfortable (aerobic) Somewhat hard (aerobic & anaerobic) Hard (anaerobic)	How you should feel with exercise – this is the target range for exercise to be effective
9 10	Very very hard Maximum exertion	Hardest you have ever worked Stop! (Overtraining)

2. The fitness parameters *(Taken from Women & the Weight Loss Tamasha)*

Let's assume that there was a workout school out there that you could attend; you'd be taught five main subjects: cardio respiratory fitness, muscular endurance, muscular strength, flexibility and body composition. You cannot do any justice to the time spent working out or the calories burnt if they do not lead to any kind of progress or learning on these five core areas of fitness.

Cardio respiratory fitness: Ability of the heart and lungs (also called as cardio-pulmonary fitness) to deliver oxygen and nutrients to working cells or muscles which are demanding them — let's say you're climbing stairs, then your leg muscles will demand more blood supply, oxygen and nutrient delivery and will need to remove or recycle waste products (like lactic acid).

Muscular strength: The greatest amount of force (maximal effort) that a muscle or a group of muscles, can exert at one time. Ever watched a cop lagao a lafa? That's muscular strength. Or when Sunny Deol says, 'Yeh dhai kilo ka haath jab padta hai to admi uthta nahi, uth jata hai' — boring exercise physiologists call it 'one rep max' but apna Bollywood describes it better.

Muscular endurance: The ability of a muscle or group of muscles to perform repeated activity over a period of time. For example, if you are moving furniture or if you are making laddoos, then you would be using your muscular endurance.

Flexibility: Ability of joints to move through their full range of motion (ROM). For example, a bowler would move his shoulder through a full range of motion before coming in to bowl.

Body composition: This refers to the fat mass that you carry as compared to the total body mass you have. For women this should be 25% or under and men 20% or under. For example, when someone says they want to look toned and not flabby, they actually mean that they would like to reduce the fat mass and increase the lean mass (bone and muscle), basically improve body composition.

Now the moral of the story is, when you make improvements on the first four parameters of fitness, it results in improvement (lowering fat mass) of the fifth parameter, that of body composition. Learning these 'subjects' or making improvements on these fitness parameters leads to an improvement in overall health, sense of wellbeing, sharpens your kinaesthetic (bodily) intelligence and yeah, improves your appearance and looks too. It also leads to perfect harmony in our hormones, leads to stable moods and puts the mind into the 'feel-good' mode, unlike the high-strung or run-down state of mind that most weight-loss plans lead to. Every time I am invited as a speaker at medical conferences or colleges, I strongly urge the medicos to use the term 'improve your body composition' or 'make improvements in strength and stamina' while advising their patients versus the often used 'just lose some weight' as a remedy to lifestyle diseases or aches and pains.

3. Muscles and TBLJ

The human body is made of different materials, broadly those that produce force — muscles — and those that don't — tendons, bones, ligaments and joints (TBLJ).

Muscles can produce force (also called as load or resistance) in three distinct ways:

1. Isometric – Force is produced without a change in the length of the muscle. For example pushing against a wall will produce no change in length of the muscles of chest, shoulders and arms but you will feel the tension nevertheless.
2. Isotonic – Force generated with change in muscle length.
    a. Concentric contraction – Force produced by shortening in the length of the muscle (mostly seen when muscles contract against the forces of gravity). For example, curling the dumbbells up will shorten the length of the bicep.

b. Eccentric contraction – Force produced by lengthening the muscle (mostly seen when muscles contract in the direction of gravity). For example, lowering the dumbbells causes lengthening of biceps in the dumbbell curl.

3. Isokinetic – Force generated by keeping the velocity of contraction constant. For example, running at a constant speed on the treadmill.

Technical note — The sliding filament theory

At a very basic level every muscle fibre is made of many tiny, smaller fibres called myofibrils. They contain even smaller structures called as actin (thin) and myosin (thick) filaments. These filaments slide in and out between each other to carry our muscle contractions and so it's called as the sliding filament theory. When the filaments slide over each other, calcium gets released from the sarcomere (functional unit of the myofibril) and ATP gets broken down to produce energy. It's this release of calcium ion that produces the energy or the current marna effect ;).

TBLJ rhymes with DDLJ and is easy to remember that way.

Tendons	• Attach muscles to bones • Transfer muscular forces across the joints that hold the bones together
Bones	• Human body has 206 bones • They act alongwith muscles as levers to transfer force • Provide support to the skeletal structure • Act as protection for internal organs • Work as calcium storage units

Ligaments	• Hold bones together in joints • Attach bones to bones
Joints	• Location at which bones connect • Allow for movement and provide mechanical support to the body • Joints differ in their mobility according to the structure. E.g. hip can move more than the knee or shoulder more than elbow
Cartilage	• Cover the ends of the bones smoothly at joints • Allow the bones to slide smoothly over each other

Exercise and physical activity have a positive effect on all of the above, increases strength, stability and flexibility, makes the human body efficient and fit to deal with life. Lack of exercise leads to deterioration of all of the above, reduces the fitness of the body and increases its fatness, thereby reducing its efficiency at leading a healthy and active life. Other than just physical factors or fitness, there is a drop in neurological, chemical, metabolical, hormonal and biological parameters too. Basically, use it or lose it.

Chapter Summary

- Move around, be active, sitting is the new smoking
- But don't confuse physical activity with exercise, both are different but important
- Just 150 minutes of exercise a week is all you need to stay fit, and keep all lifestyle disorders away
- Exercise has a dramatically beneficial effect on your heart as it becomes more efficient and stronger, especially the LV
- Of course, random workout sessions don't count, in fact they can be counterproductive
- To understand exercise, to plan your workouts, and to burn fat, you need to understand the body's energy systems
- Broadly, they are aerobic and anaerobic energy systems, and they use different types of muscles and sources of fuel
- Aerobic activities can use carbs, fat and protein as fuel while anaerobic can only use carbs in the form of muscle glycogen
- After an anaerobic activity, the body needs extra oxygen to restore all bodily functions
- This is called after-burn (or EPOC), and leads to extra calories consumed, or extra fat burned, up to 48 hours post anaerobic exercise
- Use the Borg scale to measure your effort and determine which energy system you are currently using during exercise
- It's important that your exercise program helps you make gains in all parameters of fitness — strength, endurance, flexibility and cardio-respiratory fitness

- Therefore, there is no such thing as 'best exercise', as no one exercise can train all these parameters and use all muscle fibre types and energy pathways
- You can have a favourite exercise, but for you to have a lifelong affair with it, you will need to have a wholesome workout plan
- Exercise is not for the fit, exercise makes you fit

Chapter 3

Strength Training

Strength training is the only 'medicine' you need for all lifestyle disorders, including diabetes.

An exercise we don't know much about

'You know, I don't want to become a body builder, just want to lose some weight and be able to tuck my shirt in.' 'Hmm ... no, no, don't worry, you won't...' I began, but was cut short by Sunita exclaiming, '40 pounds! This guy Vernon, my trainer, is getting me to push forty pounds on chest press! Saala mera husband se mera arms bada ho jayega.'

The one type of exercise that is riddled with controversy, fear and suspicion is weight training. Close your eyes and imagine a gym, you will see all kinds of body builders training in there. Open your eyes and you will see all kinds of regular people — college students, housewives, hi-flying executives, senior citizens trying to prevent bone loss, etc. In reality, you have to look really, really hard to find a body builder, and chances are no matter how hard you look, you won't find them. One of the reasons is that, in India, it remains a marginalized poor man's sport; most body builders can't afford to pay the kind of fees you waste every year in your eagerness to commit to making it a fitter 2014 or whatever.

And by the way, the chances of you becoming a body builder because you weight train are as high as you attaining

Samadhi because you tried savasana, or winning the Olympics 100m gold because you dashed for the Churchgate fast from platform 3 to 5. Essentially, chill! Dar ke aage jeet hai ;).

So let's get our basics right. As we learned in Chapter 2, we have the responsibility of utilizing and training our anaerobic pathways, and one of the most effective ways of doing this is called 'strength training'. Strength training is defined as use of resistance (for example, in the form of weights) to induce muscular contraction to build strength, anaerobic endurance and size of skeletal muscles. Remember the 'use it or lose it' formula? (I was contemplating on having that as the title of my book.) With age and with wealth, we start using less and less of our anaerobic pathway, and the only place where we display 'muscle' seems to be in dropping names, pulling favours and getting our kids admission in that latest / greatest / bestest school in our city. For the rest of the time, we are happy to not walk, not lift, pull, push, twist, basically very happy to not move our bodies.

Now for the diabetic capital of the world (I am talking to you) we must know that the biggest precursor of insulin resistance (high blood sugar) is loss of muscle strength. Don't ask me why your doctor didn't tell you this before. Ok, if you must ask, it's not the doctor's job to do so (the doctor's job is to give you goli ;) — it's your trainer or dietician's job. Ya, ya same dietician who told you not to strength train, uske job profile mein baithta hai. Arre baba, also don't ask why your doctor told you to walk instead of strength train. Kya bolu, your doc didn't study about energy systems, biomechanics, after-burn, etc. Now ideally, with all that money at your disposal, you should have an exercise physiologist to go to, but we have none in India. And then there are people like me, sports nutritionists who have some understanding of exercise physiology, biomechanics, kinesiology, etc., but then other than me, I don't know of anyone else. Woohooo ... so self-obsessed I am, and that is a sign of ageing. So I better run to the gym quickly and lift some weights; nothing arrests ageing like strength training does.

But then, you don't have to go to the gym to strength train; strength training only employs resistance to induce muscle contraction. So if the definition is confusing you, how about this — when you panja ladao, you strength train. When you push against a wall, the wall provides the resistance against which your pectoral muscles (chest) contract and that qualifies as strength training too. So does carrying a baby: the weight of the baby provides the resistance against which the muscles of your back, arms contract. And that's exactly why as the baby grows it gets tougher to carry, because the muscles don't have the required strength to contract against the increasing resistance (baby's increasing body weight). Walking uphill can qualify as strength training too; so will learning to lift your thighs off the floor in urdhva mukha svanasana.

Qualifying as strength training though is not enough, you must make it work for you, and it should meet your training goals (fat loss ... FAT loss — to be sung like the tune of Sachin ... SACHIN). And that's where gyms come into play with all their machines, etc., to help you train with weights lower than your body weight and with controlled movements to prevent injuries.

But for your workout to be effective, it must be planned properly. Which means you can't enter the gym and randomly declare, 'Chal aaj chest marte hai', or fool yourself into believing that twenty-five squats in the bathroom will give you a toned butt. Training after all is serious business and if you want tangible results out of it, you must be prepared to put in tangible efforts. So here goes, a crash course for you 'no time for love, no time to train' people.

But do we even need to strength train?

Wait, wait, I am jumping the gun! Am I out of my mind, wanting to teach you gym lingo when you clearly stated right at the beginning that, a) You are not the gym types b) Gyms bore you to death c) You are an outdoor person d) You are just looking to lose some weight and get a flat stomach so cardio is all you need e) You don't want muscles f) You are old and the gym is for young testosterone buzzing boys g) You are a lady and want to look like one h) You are pregnant i) You have heart trouble and / or your cholesterol is through the roof j) you are only interested in running the marathon k) You are diabetic.

Oh ho! So many reasons to not weight train! And you know, while listing your reasons, I had to refer to the alphabet chart over a hundred times coz I am dyslexic and when you blabber out so many reasons at a jet speed I just get confused. Anyway, that's not the point. I am now going to present my reasons or arguments for you to weight train and to keep it simple, I am gonna use numbers:

1) You are not the gym types 2) Gyms bore you to death 3) You are an outdoor person 4) You are just looking to lose some weight and get a flat stomach so cardio is all you need 5) You don't want muscles 6) You are old and the gym is for

young testosterone buzzing boys 7) You are a lady and want to look like one 8) You are pregnant 9) You have heart trouble and / or your cholesterol is through the roof 10) You are only interested in running the marathon 11) You are diabetic.

Really, am I so confused? No, no! My confusion was over the minute I used 1, 2, 3 instead of a, b, c, but these really are my reasons. Ok, chalo, let me give you some more reasons so that you feel it's fair and not just me copying your arguments against it as my arguments for it (and not even changing the order, so lazy!). So, how do you know you need to strength train? Read it like one of those magazine tests you are so fond of:

Do you often catch yourself doing the following:

1. Taking the lift even if you have to only go to the third or fourth floor (especially if you are a Mumbaikar, because everyone could easily climb up 4 floors until the advent of high rises and Upper Worli).
2. When you enter the lift, you rest your entire body against the wall. Or, while travelling by train, if you don't find a seat, you want to lean against the wall by the door.
3. You are driving and your building gate is closed, instead of getting out of the car to open the gate, or to look for the watchman, you just sit there and honk and stop only when you see the watchman come running towards you. While getting out of the car, you give him a piece of your mind for neglecting his 'duty'.
4. You stop your car right in front of the shop you want to visit and then murmur abuses to all the cars behind you because they are honking. I mean all these people have no manners honking at you who have double-parked but very much on the side and that too only for 5 minutes.

5. You have rolling wheels on your suitcase and have not even tried lifting it to see how much it weighs. When you hail a taxi, you expect the driver or pay a porter (after adequate bargaining, 100 nahi 50 dega, woh bhi aaj tumhara lucky day hai isliye) to load and unload it.
6. When the doorbell rings you don't move because your maid will open it and it's the kachrawali anyway.
7. You like your bean bag or like to lounge on your couch while performing difficult activities like watching TV. If the remote has been moved from its usual place, it frustrates you because now you have to 'bloody get up and look for it'.
8. You felt you were fat 5 years earlier but now when you look at those pics, you feel that you were skinny.
9. You catch yourself saying, 'But abroad you walk so much, so much exercise you get'.

Chalo deviyon aur sajjano, bhaiyo beheno, aao weight training kare, because all the above are signs of premature ageing, early degenerative diseases and lethargy and all of these are making you fat and an ideal candidate to lose out on lean body tissue or fat-free weight. The only way to keep this down and beat it is to be more self-reliant and to get strong! Strength training then is the key.

Why you must strength train

Why should you strength train? Because it uses the anaerobic pathway, therefore creates a bigger after-burn and therefore continues to burn fat even 48 hours after the workout. According to me, this is good enough reason for you to stop reading and go get a workout. But who am I kidding. You will need more than that. So let's look once again at all the excuses you came up with and see if my arguments, with explanations this time, can win you over:

1. I am not a gym person: Training in the gym, more specifically weight training, is often thought of as the preferred activity of the brain dead, but that's as far removed from the truth as Bangalore airport is from the city. The strongest proponents of weight training are some of the sharpest brains in the field of exercise physiology, kinesiology and ergonomics across the globe; these are the brains behind the training modules of Olympians. So forget all the crap you heard about training with weights, give up on this whole misconception that 'machine free' or 'free body' training is better or classier or brainier — it is not. Weight training has always been and will remain a great way to preserve youth, vigour, muscle, strength and bone density, but now it has also proved itself to be immensely useful as a heart-protecting and sugar-lowering drug. Drug? Yeah! Not all drugs need to be pharmaceuticals and prescribed by doctors!

There have been numerous studies that have proved that moderate to light weight training is as effective as hypoglycaemic drugs used in the treatment of diabetes for the first six months. After six months, the effects of weight training on blood glucose uptake and 'diabetes management' are exponentially higher than prescribed drugs. Bole toh, **weight training is way more effective in controlling and getting rid of diabetes than hypoglycaemic drugs.** But yeah, you will have to be as regular with it as you are with your medicine. And while the medicine gives you side effects like lowered sex drive, faster ageing, muscle pain, heart disease, training in the gym will give you the exact opposite — higher sex drive (irrespective of gender), anti-ageing, muscular hypertrophy and more vascularity or blood supply to the heart.

But then all this is with light or moderate strength training. This means that you should be able to perform 8 to 15 reps with good form. Now seriously, tell me how many of us would be able to use 'just body weight' to perform up to 15 reps with good technique. Most of us would tire after 2 to 4 push ups, and for the rest of us who can 'do 500 crunches or 150 sit ups', we are surely using momentum and risking our lower back to 'perform', and that is not the point of strength training. So if you are really not a gym person but still want to be a fit person, then you will need to spend at least a day in the gym per week.

***2. About gyms being boring*:** I have been training in the gym for the last 14 years without an ounce of boredom and that is because I follow the mother principle of 'progressive overload' (Chapter 6). Any training, whether in the gym or otherwise, which fails to follow this basic principle of exercise turns into a boring chore. So it's not the activity but your approach that needs to be corrected. To give you an example, when I started I would squat with 25 pounds each side on a bar of 45 pounds, do about 2 sets of 8 reps and be sore as hell for the next two days. Today, I have reached 50 pounds each side on the same 45 pound bar, my form is picture perfect, my lower back is strong, I have never sat using a back rest, and the same 2 sets and 8 reps don't make my quads sore for over a few hours. What you will learn is that strength only grows in leaps and bounds initially; later it's a struggle to keep up with the strength gains; with age, sometimes not allowing strength to drop is itself an effort, a workout in itself.

3. An outdoor person: Now this whole 'outdoor person' thing is one big facade, really. What does an outdoor person really mean? That your preferred job is that of a traffic havaldar so that all day you will spend standing outside? No na? All it means is that you want to sit in an AC office, AC car, AC theatre, etc. and then just purely out of boredom you would like to spend some time outside. Please, by all means do. Even if you commit to serious weight training in the gym, it would need as little as 2 hours per week; you are free to spend the rest of the time outdoors. Even better, walk and don't drive to the gym, outdoor ka outdoor, gym ka gym. Also, people who like being outdoors hardly ever call themselves 'an outdoor person'. Do you remember calling yourself the 'outdoor type' in school, when you spent endless time playing outside? Now just because you play one game of tennis in a club that rips you of lakhs, why call yourself that. If anything, with the increase in age, increase in weight, increase in labels and decrease in strength and flexibility, these 2 hours of gym will bless you with the ability to be outdoors for the rest of your life without being labelled an 'outdoor type'.

Remember that without strength training and without required strength in tendons, bones, ligaments and joints (TBLJ), the outdoor person in you will be stuck with a cast on one of your precious ligaments. After all, having a body means the responsibility of keeping it in good shape, and good shape comes out of good strength and not out of empty wishes.

***4. Just want to lose weight and get a flat stomach, so only cardio for me*:** Now get back to your basics, read Chapter 2 (ya, ya, again). If you just want to lose weight and sport a flat stomach, how can you possibly do that without a gain in strength? Weight training, i.e. training in the gym, not just allows you to burn calories during the period of actual exercise but also blesses you with the ability to tap into more body fat stores for the period of 36 to 48 hours post exercise. This is '**after-burn**', the period post strength training where your basal metabolic rate stays on a high. Given the bulge and circumference of our waist, our flat stomach dream will come true only with those 36 to 48 hours of fat-burning post exercise. Doing endless hours of only cardio will not lead to any after-burn and almost no gains on lean body weight. Train smart, not hard. Get it?

5. You don't want muscles: Think again. Do you want to look old and ravaged? Because that's how you will look when your muscles atrophy, that is they become smaller in size and finally destroy themselves. This is when you develop most back and knee pains, along with PMS cramps, etc. This is also what happens when you feel that you were thinner 5 years earlier than what you are today. This also translates into bye bye arms, jiggly wiggly thighs, flabby paunch, sagging butt and boobs, wrinkling face. Now would you like all that, or would you like to die young? Because if you would like to be 18 till you die, then moderate to light strength training that leads to hypertrophy of the skeletal muscle (increase in size of the muscle, along with increase in bone mineral density) is the key.

6. You are old and gymming is for the young: Hello, you are ageless and not old. The body gets old only if it doesn't keep up with strength and decreases the size of the skeletal muscle and the bone tissue. This can happen at any age, and so can anti-ageing. Training in the gym provides the body with a testosterone buzz: for men it means lower body fat, for women it means higher sex drive. Now if you are lean and sexy, who can possibly term you old?

7. You are a lady and want to look like one: Ladies, other than a higher sex drive, strength training also bestows us with strong pecs (no sagging boobs), well-rounded glutes (no more weak lower back), well-toned rectus abdominus (no more bulging midriff or fat rolling over tight jeans), sharp adductors (no more redness, infections in the inner thigh / vagina area), svelte shoulders and arms (no need to avoid that sleeveless, backless top) and stronger bone density. With all this you can easily fake your age as 24 when you are pushing 36. It allows you to period smoothly, not break out into a jungle of pimples during PMS, keeps your face radiant and taut, your fertility peaks so does your popularity. Come on now, be a lady and pump that iron.

8. You are pregnant: If you haven't strength trained before getting pregnant, then there is a good chance that you are pregnant thanks to some 'technique' and not just plain sex. Ok, sorry, no more extrapolation of facts but here goes — training during pregnancy is safe and in fact recommended. It reduces labour time, provides more oxygen and circulation to the foetus, and your baby knows that mama is a strong woman ☺. Wait, a well-rounded butt (muscular butt) is a marker of the baby's intelligence and has been linked to high scores on tests. Now I have your attention, mommies?

9. You have heart and cholesterol issues: I have a conspiracy theory. Pharma companies and hospitals have compromised mainstream media to not carry 'news' of how strength training improves the efficiency of the left ventricle (makes circulation more efficient and effortless), even though this is something that every bacha kacha with minimum exposure to exercise physiology knows, understands and appreciates. Heart is also a muscle, and with increase in strength of voluntary muscles, the involuntary muscles like the heart, intestines, etc., grow in strength, vascularity and efficiency too. Yeah and with decrease in skeletal muscle size, the heart atrophies too, leading to blood pressure, smaller stroke volume, higher resting heart rate, all in all, a ready-made case for heart disease and hyperlipidaemia. And this, in the age of 'technology and drugs', is a fast growing commodity, something on which the 'health industry' feeds. Samjha kya?

A heart that works more efficiently also translates to smooth kidney function, so less vulnerability to stress and unreasonable rage, less chances of bloating, less chances of jet-lagging and improved chances of a drug-free, stress-free life. Like that?

As for cholesterol, nothing like weight training and its added advantage of after-burn to bring that LDL, VLDL down and HDL up. Cholesterol is a problem only when the LDL and VLDL along with triglycerides are not being utilized sensibly by the body. As a matter of training response or adaptation (expect this to set in about 12 weeks post consistent exercise), the body learns to preferentially use the triglycerides and cholesterol and to spare the muscle glycogen (muscle fuel stores) for its metabolic needs. No cholesterol lowering drug can do that for you.

10. You only want to run the marathon: Well, then take a leaf out of the elite runners' book — strength train 2 to 3 days a week in the off season, and once a week during season. That's why they run those 42 km in less than 2½ hours, while you struggle to finish the 21 km in that much time. Runners are made in the gym and run on the road. Remember the basics that heart and lungs are infinitely stronger than tendons, bones, ligaments and joints? What does running really jar, the TBLJ or the heart? The stronger the skeletal tissue, the stronger, faster and leaner the runner. Now come on, don't just gulp down the pasta on the night before the marathon to run like a pro; to run like a pro, join a gym. (More in the cardio chapter.)

11. You have diabetes: Boy, you really are stuck with your diabetes sob story. I wrote about diabetes already in the first point, but here is some more gyaan. So, Interleukin-6 is an exercise responsive cytokine that muscle cells produce and release in response to contraction. And now because I am not your high funda endocrinologist or the dietician who sits outside his office with a white coat and attitude to match, I will tell you what this actually means. Don't worry, mere paas bahut time hai! ;) Btw, all this jargon bores me too and I believe jargon is fattening. But since we are in the business of keeping fit, here goes:

Cytokine: cyto – cell, kinos – movement. So Cytokines are (protein-like) substances that certain cells produce which send local signals and have an effect on other cells of your body. They are similar to hormones in the body. You can think of them as the language that your body cells use to communicate with each other.

So IL-6 is one of the many cytokines in your body that is released by our muscles in response to exercise. There is now increasing evidence and buzz in the biochemistry corridors that this may be a crucial link to controlling blood sugars and may even lead to the muscle cell being qualified as an endocrine organ. But lab and academic buzz apart, this is what it will do for you:

- Modulate / regulate glucose production
- Increase glucose uptake by cells (thereby stabilizing blood sugar levels)
- Increase GLUT-4 (molecule responsible for transporting glucose) translocation in a manner similar to insulin
- Improve functioning of the beta cells of pancreas (the organ responsible for producing insulin and glucagon which together keep your blood sugars stable)
- Work like an insulin mimicker

Short mein bole toh, there is increasing evidence that **strength training is crucial to control the 'epidemic' of diabetes.** The evidence always existed but now newer pathways are getting documented and accumulated in research to prove what common sense always knew — exercise is non-negotiable, strength training is not just safe but recommended, working out not just reduces body fat but improves cellular function and in turn prevents every possible lifestyle disorder / disease, diabetes included. Abhi when all this research will lend itself to practice, is something you can decide.

Strength training in practice — from knowing to doing

Anyway, I am assuming that you are now adequately brainwashed and are now seriously going to gym, I mean you really want to. With all this science you can't turn your back on it anymore, khali time ka lafda hai. So I am gonna help you plan your strength training routine. It takes very little time you know — and you can start with as little as an hour every week. The most important thing that you need to remember about strength training, however, is intensity. Just going to the gym and doing time pass activities like running around with a weight in hand, or doing endless crunches, or using very light weights and working on only selective muscles, etc., will not lead to any of the benefits of an anaerobic workout. A gym workout needs to be planned properly (common sense again is the golden rule), and let's look at how to do that:

1. Common strength training terms
2. Rules to plan the sequence in a strength training workout
3. Designing your workout and sample training plans
4. Guidelines to make progress

1. Common terms used in the gym

Set: The number of times you perform a certain exercise is called a set.

Reps: The number of times you lift the weight is called repetitions or reps.

Form: The correct technique to lift the weight or to contract muscles against resistance.

Rep range: Deciding the number of times you will lift a certain weight for all the sets. Typically the rep range is used to classify training as either 'light' or 'heavy', and not the weight you are lifting.

Between 3 to 5 reps per set is heavy

8 to 10 reps per set is moderate
12 to 15 reps per set is light
15 to 20 reps per set is very light

Split: The pattern in which body parts are 'split' for training in a week. For example, if you train the upper body one day and lower body on another, you are on a 2-day split. If you are training full body together once a week, you are on a 1-day split.

Technical note — Heavy, light or moderate

It's not the weight but the energy pathway that is employed to lift a weight and its associated oxygen debt and lactic acid production that qualifies a training session as heavy, moderate, light or very light. Light (or very light) weight training involves contracting muscles up to 20 reps with good technique; this uses the aerobic pathway (as the load is light) and creates little or no oxygen debt. So even if you lifted 100 kilos on the leg press but lifted it with good technique for 20 reps and without reaching fatigue, it is very light weight training, irrespective of your gender.

Heavy weight training, on the other hand, is when you can lift only 3 to 5 reps with good form. Most of us beginners reach that point with as little as 2 or 5 pounds on the side laterals that train the middle deltoid (shoulder). So 5 pounds may seem 'light' but it has employed the anaerobic pathway for contracting the muscles involved and is therefore 'heavy' due to EPOC and other factors. This same 5 pounds on a lunge could allow you to do 20 reps and therefore qualify as light weight training as it has employed the aerobic pathway for the muscles involved.

---

2. Rules to plan the correct weight training sequence

There are certain rules that need to be followed so that your time spent in the gym is most effective. These are:

1. Warm-up should be specific to the main workout
2. Exercise should recruit maximum number of muscle fibres
3. Duration of workout should never exceed 60 minutes

Based on these rules, a correct sequence of strength or weight training has been evolved which is followed world over, though I'm not sure if it's being followed in the gym you go to. Now, here is the thing: if you don't want to get into details of these rules and how the sequence developed and just want to get on with the planning bit, skip straight to page 77 for the summary. Otherwise, read on.

The three basic rules to plan a weight training sequence:

Rule 1 – Specific warm-ups

A common mistake in gyms is either a complete lack of warm-up or doing a completely non-specific warm-up. A complete lack of warm-up will very obviously jolt the joints and use momentum versus technique to bring about movement, which will lead to an injury if not now then definitely by the next session. There is basic awareness nowadays, so most people do a 'warm-up', but in a really time pass manner. Some common examples:

- Walking / jogging for 10 to 20 minutes on the treadmill before performing weight training exercises (ya, that's wrong even if you are doing legs and not upper body).
- Running 5 or 20 times or whatever random number

your coach barked out to you today around the tennis court before picking up your racquet.

- Number 3, reminder to Ms Rujuta. Madam, focus on weight training and leave this tennis-phennis cribs to another time.

Ok, so only weight training example, then. The right warm-up allows the blood flow to move through the specific muscle groups and warms up the specific joints that will be trained that day. Other than saving time, this saves another precious entity, muscle glycogen. So on a day when you squat, you should warm up using less than 50% of the weight you will squat with; same goes for back or chest. And once you have warmed up on the multiple-joint exercises, you don't need to warm up when you move to single-joint exercises.

Follow these instructions for a correct warm-up:

i. Perform a warm-up set of 12 to 15 reps before starting your training
ii. Use 50% of the main workout weight
iii. Rest for 30 seconds to 3 minutes before starting the main workout set

This leads to muscles and joints being warmed up with the exact mechanics that will be performed on the workout set. It reduces chances of using momentum to lift weights, allows you to lift maximum weight in the main set, makes muscles less susceptible to injury and provides for a sort of dress rehearsal for the breathing and motor skill.

Rule 2 – Maximum muscle fibre recruitment

This is the golden principle of weight training — the more muscle fibres you recruit, the more you can lift. The more you lift, the more calories you burn both during exercise and as after-burn.

To recruit maximum muscle fibres, the chosen exercise should:

iv. Involve maximum number of joints, as moving through more joints means recruitment of more muscle fibres versus moving through a single joint.

v. Train larger muscle groups before the smaller muscle groups as they have a higher ability to employ muscle fibres.

Other than training bigger muscle groups first and movement through multiple joints, there is another factor that influences the 'muscle fibre recruitment' — it's called the 'substrate availability', or in simple words, the fuel available to fire (employ) these muscle fibres.

Fuel for strength training

Now, as we know, weight training uses the anaerobic system, more specifically the glycogen lactic acid system. The muscles contract and therefore perform exercises using their stored glycogen stores. Muscle glycogen is not just short in supply but takes a long time to replenish once its stores are exhausted. With regular exercise our body adapts and responds by increasing its ability to store muscle glycogen. But for beginners or even trained athletes, the sequence of exercise is of paramount importance because you don't want to run out of fuel before you reach the main task or perform the big calorie-burning exercises.

This fuel limitation has led to one more instruction being added to make your exercise more efficient, both in burning calories as well as improving on the strength and bone mineral density. This is:

vi. Perform higher intensity before lower intensity exercises.

If you look at the reference table for strength training (on page 80) and apply these rules, then you would work out in the following order — legs, back, chest, shoulders, arms. And within legs you would prioritize multiple joints exercises like squats before leg extension. And with the chest you would chest press (higher intensity, more exhausting) before doing the flies. And with the back you would want to do a bent over row, which is done using 'free weights' like the barbell, and is of higher intensity, before doing a seated row. Use of machines reduces the intensity (and so the exhaustion) even if the muscle group employed is the same as in the example of bent over row and seated row.

Technical note — Correct technique

Essential to performing any weight training workout is the correct technique or the form. This means:

- Allowing joints to move through their full range of motion (ROM)
- Not using momentum to create movement

This follows from the maximum muscle recruitment principle. A muscle, which is fatigued by the use of single-joint exercises, will not be able to allow the joints to move through the full range of motion in a multi-joint exercise. For example, after contracting and fatiguing the quads through leg extensions, the legs will not be able to contract the quads through the full range of motion in a squat or lunge or even step ups. This will not just limit the efficiency of the squat or the multi-joint exercise, but will pose a risk to the joint involved. Thoughtless exercise behaviour that pays no attention to the science behind exercise is the leading cause of gym injuries, mostly to the poor little TBLJ, sometimes straining the muscle too.

This whole prioritizing of exercises is not just to make optimum use of glycogen but also because the sequence of exercise has a profound effect on fat-burning.

After-burn

When larger muscles are employed using multiple joints and the intensity is kept challenging or high, then it not just results in maximum calories burnt in that one hour of exercise but it also gives you more after-burn. After-burn is when the body, at rest, burns calories at a higher rate post exercise as compared to what it would normally have (Chapter 2).

A very important consequence of after-burn or EPOC is that the anaerobic pathways can take up to 48 hours to recover, so never plan weight training or sprinting sessions on consecutive days. Without adequate recovery, no anabolism and therefore no fat loss can take place. Also, what you should keep in mind is that lactic acid, which is a by-product of anaerobic metabolism, can be used as a fuel by the aerobic pathway. **It makes sense then to plan an aerobic workout on the day after the anaerobic;** it helps achieve two things: the aerobic pathway can use lactic acid as a fuel and lactic acid can get used up quickly (removed from muscle), leading to better recovery from the anaerobic workout.

So you should pay close attention to the exercise sequence, not just what you do on any given day, but what you plan to do a day prior or after the exercise. So let's add one more to the instructions:

vii. Allow for adequate recuperation (two days at least) between two weight training sessions (to allow the body to repay oxygen debt, re-synthesize glycogen and repair wear and tear to the muscle tissue).

This rule is applicable even if you are training two different body parts in consecutive sessions.

Technical note — Soreness or DOMS

Glycogen, the fuel that is used during exercise, provides the energy for muscle contraction by breaking itself down and creating a by-product called 'lactic acid'. With accumulation of lactic acid in the muscle, the muscle experiences fatigue and beyond a certain concentration of lactic acid, the muscle will refuse to contract or take part in exercise. Which means that even if the muscle has the required strength, in the presence of a certain concentration of lactic acid, it will be unable to perform the task at hand. It is exactly this lactic acid concentration in the blood that leads to what is called as 'soreness' in the muscles, the meetha meetha dard that you feel the next day after exercise. In weight training lingo, this is called 'delayed onset of muscular soreness' (DOMS). So let's say you trained your legs on Monday, on Tuesday your legs revolt even when you want to get off the chair or sit on one. It's not that your quads don't have the required strength to get off the chair or your hamstrings have lost the ability to lower you onto the chair, but they hurt and show unwillingness to perform these activities. What should you do then? Rest? No, that would make it worse. The thing to do then, is more activity, more specifically an aerobic workout, a light jog, walk or cycling for half an hour. This is because the muscles, liver, heart and even kidney tissue in the presence of oxygen can use up the lactic acid.

Rule 3 – Duration not more than 60 minutes

Well, actually, with the glycogen stores most of us have, we will run out of fuel in as little as 30 minutes. So other than following all the rules above, we must remember that once the glycogen stores are over, then the body will burn its proteins to keep up with the exercise. This will lead to both a drop in exercise intensity and a higher risk of injury. Wasting protein or burning it for metabolic processes like producing energy for muscle fibre contraction is the exact opposite of the goal of weight training.

More than 60 minutes spent in the gym is also a major factor in the drop-out rate. Given our 'lifestyles' — caught in traffic, caught in lifts, caught in relationships, caught in jobs, etc. — we shouldn't be caught wasting muscle protein or breaking down amino acids in the gym. This leads to breakdown of more muscle than our lifestyle allows us to repair or recover from. Soon this leads to the well-documented, well-experienced behaviour of, 'I paid for the full year last year but didn't go beyond a week'. It's best to keep exercise to an hour, including warm-up, workout sets and cool down, and perhaps even the drive back home if you live close by. This will improve exercise compliance and lead to reduction in guilt + body fat, again brought about by the exercise compliance. So, because you have limited time for your workout session, use these rules to help you structure it:

viii. In one gym session perform about 8 to 10 sets (excluding warm-up) that train major muscle groups.
ix. Perform 8 to 15 reps per set, with good form and to a point of fatigue (fatigue is reached when you know you can't do another repetition with the same weight without compromising on form).
x. Use both multi- and single-joint exercises.

Technical note — Exercise and immune system

Typically, any time there's cellular damage either because of virus or a wound, there is an associated immune response. However, the response to the different types of injuries is quite similar. There's an increase in white blood cells, natural killer (NK) cells and T-cells (fighter of infections).

Now believe it or not, exercise is a physical stressor and has an immune-suppressing response. This is especially true if the duration of exercise is longer than 60 minutes. Spending longer than 60 minutes in the gym either at one go or by doing things like working out twice a day decreases the number of NK and T-cells. This effect lasts for up to 72 hours post exercise, making you susceptible to infections, flu, etc. The exact opposite of getting fit.

Summary of rules to plan your strength training workout:

Basic rules	Instructions for sequence of strength training workout	Examples / Comments
1. Specific warm-ups	i. Perform warm up set of 12-15 reps before workout set ii. Use 50% of the main workout weight iii. Rest for 30 seconds to 3 minutes before starting main workout set	– Warm-up allows the blood flow to move through the specific muscle groups and warms up the specific joints that will be trained
2. Maximum muscle fibre recruitment	iv. Train large muscle groups before small muscle groups v. Train multiple joints before single joints vi. Perform higher intensity before lower intensity exercises vii. Allow for adequate recuperation between two weight-training sessions	– Back before biceps – Squats before leg extensions – Chest press before flies – After-burn and recovery continues for 36-48 hours after weight-training session

Basic rules	Instructions for sequence of strength training workout	Examples / Comments
3. Duration should not exceed 60 minutes	viii. Perform about 8-10 sets in total (excluding warm-up) that train major muscle groups ix. Perform 8-15 reps per set, with good form and to a point of fatigue x. Use both multi- and single-joint exercises	– Glycogen stores don't last beyond 60 minutes, usually 30 minutes – After glycogen stores are over, body starts breaking down muscle protein

Least important, most seen

The 'concentration' curl, where the guy sits on the bench smiling at the camera, his elbow flexed, a dumbbell in his hand moving towards the shoulder, is one of the most commonly seen photographs of 'weight training'. The truth is this 'popular' exercise is missing from the routine of most serious weight trainers! The reason is that it's amongst the smallest muscles, so it's performed fewer times a month as compared to the big muscle exercises like squats, dead lifts and chest press. Now these don't get photographed too much because they make for poor picture composition and you can't look pretty or attractive performing these exercises, let alone smile and gaze flirtatiously at the camera. So you see a guy with dole-shole and a paunch to match, then he belongs to the category that trains the smaller muscles more than the bigger muscles (and I say don't date that kind, date the kind with a flat stomach and bulging triceps). Same goes for women who complain of 'bulking up' post weight training. They are resting the big calorie burners (big muscles — legs, back, chest) and are doing the favourite and most photographed female exercise — the lunge — with pretty pink dumbbells that the model curls to her shoulders as she poses for the pic.

Pictures may say a thousand words, but not the fitness photographs. Always remember that they are exceptions to the rule.

3. Designing your workout and sample training plans

Our body can be roughly divided into the upper body and lower body. Everything hips and lower is considered the 'lower body' or 'legs' in gym lingo. Everything above the hips is 'upper body'. The 'upper body' is further divided into pushing and pulling muscles. The pushing muscles are chest, anterior deltoid (front portion of your shoulder) and triceps (the back of your arm), and the pulling ones are your back, posterior deltoid (back of the shoulder) and biceps.

So, based on this, you can split your workout per week as:

1-day split: Full body workout once a week

2-day split: Upper body one day and lower body on the other

3-day split: Lower body one day, pushing muscles second day and pulling muscles third day

For each of the muscle groups there are certain exercises you can perform in the gym. The most common exercises, along with muscle types, the number of joints involved, etc., are presented for easy reference in the table below.

THE reference table for strength training

Muscle group (from big to small)	Exercise(s)	Free / assisted on machine	Joints involved	Compound / Isolation
1. Legs – Note that compound exercises on legs use all the muscles of the lower body as well as the core.				
Glutes (hip muscle)	Squats Lunges Step ups	Free, done with a barbell on shoulders	Hip Lower back Knee Ankle	Involves multiple joints to flex (bend) and extend (open out) simultaneously, so compound.
	Leg press	Machine with plates / stack	Machine reduces involvement of lower back but hip, knee, ankle active	Compound
Quads (front of the thigh)	Leg extension	Machine	Knee	Isolation
Hamstring (back of the thigh)	Stiff leg dead lift	Free with barbell in hand	Hip & knee	Compound
	Leg curl	Machine	Knee	Isolation

Gastroc and soleus (calf muscle)	Calf raises Toe raises	Free with BB/DB or with machine	Ankle	Isolation
Adductor (outer thigh) Abductor (inner thigh)	Adductor Abductor	Mostly machines or done lying down (all side-kick varieties)	Hip	Isolation
2. Back				
Erector spinae (lower back, the muscle that runs parallel to the spine)	Dead lift	Similar to the squat but BB held in hand vs on shoulders.	Lower back Hip Knee Ankle	Compound
	Back extension	Lying on floor/bench	Lower back	Isolation
Lats (middle back)	Bent over row 1 arm DB row T bar rows Lat pull down Seated row Pull ups*	Machine and/or free *mostly on machine as most of us too weak to do 8 -12 reps	Back Shoulder Elbow	Compound – moves through many joints
Traps (upper back)	Shrugs	Free with DB / BB	Shoulder blades, Shoulder	Isolation

<table>
<tr><td colspan="5">3. Chest - Sometimes also called as upper & lower pec to mean upper or lower part of chest.</td></tr>
<tr><td>Pecs
(Chest
muscles)</td><td>Chest
press
Incline/
Decline /
Flat DB or
BB press</td><td>Machine
Done on a
bench</td><td>Chest
Shoulder
(front)
Elbow</td><td>Compound –
moves through
many joints</td></tr>
<tr><td></td><td>Push up</td><td>Free but
most not
strong to do
8-12 with
good form</td><td>Involves lower
back & other
core muscles
too</td><td>Compound</td></tr>
<tr><td></td><td>Flies</td><td>Can be done
both free
using DB or
machine</td><td>Shoulder</td><td>Isolation – uses
primarily one
joint</td></tr>
<tr><td colspan="5">4. Shoulders or Deltoid – has 3 heads or parts – back (posterior), middle & front (anterior) of the shoulder. Every upper body exercise will involve the deltoid. Training the back involves the p.delt & chest the a. delt. Depending on the choice of back & chest exercise, shoulder involvement varies.</td></tr>
<tr><td>Posterior
delt (back)

Middle
delt
(middle)
Anterior
delt (front)</td><td>Rev fly

Side
laterals

Front
raises
Overhead-
presses*</td><td>Free &
machine

Free &
machine

Free &
machine</td><td>Shoulder</td><td>Largely
isolation
exercises –
involves only
one joint

*Overhead
press is
compound as
it uses elbows
too along with
shoulders</td></tr>
</table>

5. Arms - Every upper body exercise will involve arms. The back involves the bicep & chest the tricep.				
Tricep (back of the arm)	DB extension	Free	Elbow	Isolation
	Pushdown	Free or machine	Shoulder Elbow Wrist – small involvement	Compound
Bicep (front of the arm)	Curls of all types	Free / machine	Elbow	Isolation

Below is a suggested set of guidelines that you can use to design your gym workout:

- If you have never worked out before, start with a 1-day split
- After 10 workouts, if you are up to it, move to a 2-day split
- After 12 weeks of the 2-day split, move to a 3-day split. If you don't feel like it, continue with the 2-day split
- Weight training twice a week is extremely efficient for making gains in strength, BMD and loss of body fat.
- If you feel like it, you can also do:

  Week 1 – Full body (1 day)
  Week 2 – Upper body and lower body (2 days)
  Week 3 – Lower body (1 day)
  Week 4 – Upper body and lower body (2 days)
  Week 5 – Upper body (1 day)
  Week 6 – Upper body and lower body (2 days)

This way you can make twice-a-week investments every alternate week but keep up with a routine without getting bored.

Sample strength training plans

1-day split OR Beginner's plan

Exercise	Target muscle group	Sets	Reps
Leg press	Quads, glutes, hamstrings	2	12-15
Leg extension	Quads	1	12-15
Leg curl	Hamstrings	1	12-15
Lat pull down	Lats (back), traps, post. delt, biceps	1-2	12-15
Seated row	Lats (back), traps, post. delt, biceps	1	12-15
Dumbbell / Bar press	Pecs, ant. delt, triceps	2	12-15
Pec dec / fly	Pecs	1	12-15
Side laterals	Middle deltoid	1	12-15

2-day split OR Intermediate plan

Exercise	Target muscle group	Sets	Reps
Lower body			
Squats	Glutes, quads, hams, adductor, abductor, calf	2	10-12
Leg press	Quads, glutes, hamstrings	2	10-12
Leg extension	Quads	1-2	10-12

Leg curl	Hamstrings	1-2	10-12
Calf raises	Gastroc	2	10-12
Upper body			
Lat pull down	Lats (back), traps, post. delt, biceps	1-2	10-12
Seated row	Lats (back), traps, post. delt, biceps	1-2	10-12
Hyper extension	Erector spinae	1	10-12
Dumbbell / Bar press	Pecs, ant. deltoid, triceps	2	10-12
Pec dec / fly	Pecs	1-2	10-12
Side laterals	Middle deltoid	1 -2	10-12
Dumbbell curl	Biceps	1	10-12
Tricep push down	Triceps	1	10-12

3-day split OR Advanced plan

Exercise	Target muscle group	Sets	Reps
Lower body			
Squats	Glutes, quads, hams, adductor, abductor, calves	2	8-10
Lunges	Glutes, quads, hams, adductor, abductor, calves	2	8-10
Leg extension	Quads	1	8-10

Stiff leg deadlift	Glutes and hamstrings	2	8-10
Leg curl	Hamstrings	1-2	8-10
Standing Calf raises	Gastroc	1-2	8-10
Seated calf raises	Soleus	1-2	8-10
Pulling muscles – back, post. delt, biceps			
Barbell row	Lats (back), traps, post. delt, biceps	2	8-10
Lat pull down	Lats (back), traps, post. delt, biceps	2	8-10
Shrugs	Traps	2	8-10
Reverse pec deck	Post. delt	2	8-10
Barbell curl	Biceps	2	8-10
Hammer curl	Biceps	1	8-10
Pushing muscles – Chest, ant. delt, triceps			
Incline / decline DB press	Pecs, ant. delt, tricep	2	8-10
Flat machine press OR seated chest press	Pecs, ant. delt, tricep	1	8-10
Pec dec / fly	Pecs	2	8-10
Overhead DB press	Pecs, ant. delt, tricep (more involement of ant. delt)	1	8-10
Side lateral DB	Middle deltoid	2	8-10
Cable push down	Triceps	1	8-10
DB extension	Triceps	1	8-10

Note: Exercise list is indicative and not exhaustive. Exercises to be performed in the order mentioned.

Choosing the right trainer

I recommend, very strongly, working with a qualified trainer for the first 6 to 12 sessions to learn the basics of right technique and even a little know-how of the gym equipment, like where to adjust the seat based on your height for a leg curl / chest press, etc. However, never ever work with a trainer who is more than willing to be just a spotter, counting for you, waiting on you, adjusting your seat, wiping the sweat of your brow and putting the dumbbell back on the rack for you. All this can be done by a friend in exchange for your company in the gym and perhaps even in return for the same favour. Get a trainer who cares about timing, yours as well as hers / his, teaches you to work out on your own, is well-versed with the terms that you know exist in exercise physiology based on this book (full of myself, full of myself again), charges above Rs 6,500 per month, and doesn't let you 'make up' lost sessions. Look for a taskmaster, for a professional. And once they charge Rs 10,000 upwards, ensure that they are registered and provide you with a service tax number, no not because you are willing to shell out 12 or 10% extra based on Chidambaram's mood, but because trainers who pay taxes and have their registrations in place are more likely to stay focused and learn and update themselves with the latest in physiology and training.

4. Guidelines to progress in your workout

Making progress is almost as important as starting to work out, so:

1. Do not attempt to increase both weight and reps in the same workout session. If you increased reps one week, then in week 2 you could increase the weight and week 3 increase sets. Increasing more than one component of training in the same week risks both injuries and early dropouts.
2. At any point of time, if you can lift a weight comfortably for the suggested number of reps, then it's time to increase the weight.
3. Weight may be increased by as little as 2½ pounds at a time.
4. If an increase in weight leads to decrease of reps below 6 or compromises on form, use this example to modify your plan:

   Example: You can do 15 reps of 10 pounds on a dumbbell curl, but the next dumbbell in the gym is 15 pounds and that decreases your reps to less than 6.

   – Do 3 reps with 15 pounds and the rest with 10 pounds.
   – Over a period of time the muscles will learn to push 15 pounds up to 8 reps.
   – Once this happens you can stop performing the remaining reps with 10 pounds and officially graduate to 15 pounds.
   – Continue on 15 pounds till 12 reps is a challenge.
   – When the body adapts and you can do more than 15 reps easily on 15 pounds, look for the 20 pound dumbbell and repeat.

Just like there are endless books on meditation but nothing can give you even a glimpse of what the real thing is, I can endlessly 'break down' weight training exercises, but this book cannot teach you what a session in the gym will. A man after all is what he does and not what he thinks and much less what he reads ;).

Meal planning for strength training

Eating right is more crucial for weight training than any other form of exercise, because weight training leads to maximum metabolic and biochemical changes in the body. For starters, there's the fact that it utilizes the precious entity of muscle glycogen, which can take days to replenish itself. Then there's the oxygen debt that needs to be repaid, which leads to accelerated fat metabolism up to 48 hours post exercise. And last but not least, there is the free radical effect, the by-products of metabolism, basically chemically unstable molecules which can cause cellular damage, take the edge out of your exercise and even lead to ageing. So before we get into meal planning, let's look at the catabolic and anabolic process and hormonal changes that occur due to weight training

Cortisol and Insulin — Break down and make up

There are two hormones that are the cornerstones of meal plans before, during and after weight training. These are the catabolic hormone **cortisol**, and the anabolic hormone **insulin**. Popular literature projects both as some sort of villain, but they are essential for weight training. Cortisol's major function is to provide fuel for the working muscle group. However, post exercise, if cortisol levels are not kept in check, then the entire anabolic (anti-ageing) benefit brought about by exercise is lost. **Mindless training beyond an hour and**

improper meal planning post exercise are the two main reasons that people 'stagnate' or 'plateau' in their workout routines. An elevated level of cortisol — which prevents the re-synthesis of glycogen and breaks down more protein than the body can repair — brings about this plateau phenomenon and negates any benefit that an exercise program can offer.

Immediately post exercise, our muscle cells have heightened insulin sensitivity. Which means that we have a brilliant window of opportunity for 45 minutes post exercise, where we can push maximum nutrients into our muscle cells. A meal which comprises water, carbs, protein, fat, vitamins and minerals that leads to a surge in insulin levels can a) arrest muscle breakdown, b) increase the speed of glycogen re-synthesis, c) increase glucose uptake by the muscles, d) increase the muscle contractile protein which increases both size and strength of the muscle tissue, e) increase the blood flow to the muscles which improves both nutrient delivery as well as removal of waste like CO_2 and lactic acid from the muscles and f) brings down the cortisol levels, thereby helping the body maintain its immune function.

With this understanding of cortisol and insulin, let's look at the pre- and post-workout meal options.

Crunches before the party for that flat stomach

Now don't tell me you haven't tried this only to notice, much to your disappointment, that the stomach bulged out like a balloon out of your tight tee or LBD. So to ensure that this doesn't happen at the next party, you crunched 500 times versus your usual 100, and that evening the stomach bulged out 500 times more. Finally you gave up and didn't do any crunches just before a party, and voila, the stomach looked flatter than ever. Chalo, let me tell you why that happens.

When there is tissue damage, whether exercise-related or otherwise, the body's acute inflammatory response gets activated. Within hours of damage, special cells called neutrophils migrate to the site of damage (your abs in this case) and remove tissue debris. (The neutrophil response can last for many hours post exercise and is also considered one of the factors that lead to muscle soreness.) This process causes inflammation (bloating), swelling and further tissue damage. More crunches mean more tissue damage, which means more bloating and swelling, which in turn will cause more tissue damage. All in all, you are breaking more than you can repair, and all it leads to is a flabbier stomach. So don't make a big deal out of your stomach, **just focus on the real DEAL — a wholesome Diet, Exercise and Lifestyle;** the stomach will take care of itself.

Pre-and post-workout meals

Planning both pre-and post-exercise meals is critical to getting 'results' — that sculpted look comes much more from what you eat before and after exercise than just exercise itself. So here goes:

Pre-workout: A fruit (local, seasonal) is always a good option, especially if you are training first thing in the morning or leaving from office and going to the gym before you head home. A gap of 15 to 20 minutes between the fruit and the warm-up set is all you need. If you are the type who goes to the gym post breakfast or lunch, then a gap of 60 to 100 minutes is good. Avoid meat before the workout as it is devoid of fibre and takes longer to leave your GI tract than a vegetarian meal. Food in the stomach while exercising will restrict blood flow to the working muscle group, thereby reducing its ability to recruit optimum muscle, which will hamper the efficiency of the exercise. However, if you would like to add protein to your meals before working out, then just a wholesome meal of poha / paratha / dosa / rice-dal will do the trick, or you can even add 10g (half scoop) of whey protein with your fruit or meal.

Post-workout: A post-workout meal is ideally something you carry to the gym and that you eat the minute you have cooled down. So you are most likely to finish with a single joint / small group exercise, then do your stretches, check that you have placed all dumbbells / barbells back on the rack and you are ready to eat.

There are 4 R's of a post workout meal that you must follow very strictly if you want to get the most out of your workout. The whole point of eating right before and after a workout is that you look 'worked out' when you are wearing your regular clothes, shirt-pant, salwar-kurta, jeans-tee shirt, saree, skirt-top, etc. Too often, in spite of 'so much I workout', all that shows in your regular clothes is a fat stomach and a flat butt and it's only when you wear 'workout clothes', like a white tee shirt and shorts or black tights and bright pink tee, that people know that you gym. You can change that by just timing your meals right.

More and more research in sports nutrition is focused on how 'timing' of fuel (meals) affects performance. So not just the 4 R's but also the 4 hours post exercise is crucial to the glycogen replenishment that will take place in the muscle tissue.

This will influence everything else involved, from the way you rebuild lost muscle tissue to the strength gains you make, the bone mineral density you build and the fat burning that you will achieve and sustain. Pay close attention to this now:

The 4 R's of post-workout nutrition

1. *R – Rehydrate*: Have a glass of water to quench your thirst, and then have another one. Remember that thirst is not a reliable signal during and post exercise; the body is in a dehydrated condition post a workout, so even if there's no thirst signal present or even if it vanishes after a sip of water, continue to drink. The water temperature can be room temperature or cooled but never hot or warm.
2. *R – Replenish*: Eating a fruit like banana or having a boiled potato will replenish your glycogen stores and your blood sugar levels. The glycaemic index, digestibility, taste and potassium stores all go in favour of the banana and potato. They provide for a light, easy and healthy meal that can quickly replenish the glycogen stores without overloading the gastro-intestinal system or disrupting the blood flow to the worked-out muscles.
3. *R – Repair*: A good protein shake made out of whey protein can provide the body with all the required amino acids to carry out its repair work and arrest further tissue damage. Whey protein is liquid in nature, with a ratio of essential to non-essential amino acids that makes it easy to digest and assimilate, and it can carry out its repair work without hampering the post-workout metabolic environment in the body. Whey protein scores on another count: in its levels of branched chain amino acids (BCAAs). These are

a group of three essential amino acids that are sacrificed or burnt down during periods of intense exercise or stress. These BCAAs also synthesize the non-essential amino acid glutamine, which looks after the immune system in the body. When BCAAs get broken down, the glutamine levels drop and with it the body's immune function takes a beating. The BCAAs along with glutamine and other essential amino acids also work at keeping the insulin sensitive and allow the body to improve its fat-burning response. (More about whey protein shakes at the end of the chapter.)

4. *R – Recover*: The free radicals generated during exercise (or any physical activity) are chemically unstable and cause a lot of damage that can come in the way of the body's recovery from exercise. Antioxidants are basically molecules that can donate an electron to these free radicals and stop them from further oxidation or breakdown. Most vitamins like C, E, A and minerals like selenium, zinc and chromium are well known for their antioxidant effect. What's more, selenium, zinc and chromium work at keeping the insulin efficient, even mimicking the insulin response and aiding the body's recovery from exercise. This obviously then is the time that your body is most primed to make use of your antioxidant / anti-ageing / skin-hair-nail supplements. Even if you don't have one by that name, just separate pills for vitamins C, E and beta-carotene along with a mineral supplement for selenium, zinc and chromium will do the trick and be less of a load on your wallet too.

The 4 R's need to get done within the first 45 minutes after exercise — actually better if you finish within the first 20 minutes only. I get all my clients who are beginners with weight training, or those who come to me because they have plateaued, or the ones who have special needs like pregnancy, diabetes, rheumatoid arthritis, BP, etc. to finish the 4 R's within the first 20 minutes itself. It's only the experienced who actually have the option of eating within 45 minutes instead of 20 (although they are most likely to eat within the first 5 minutes). You see, post exercise the blood glucose levels are low, actually you are in a state of hypoglycaemia and that is a precursor for high cortisol levels. I don't like my clients roaming around on high cortisol levels that wipe out the anabolic effects of exercise. Moreover, the hypoglycaemia, along with the natural surge in insulin levels, can lead to insulin insensitivity over a period of time. This means that just because you delayed your post-workout meal, you developed central obesity and eventually diabetes. That's not what you worked out for, you can develop that even without exercise, so just time those meals right and have the 4 R's immediately after working out.

The 4 hours post exercise

After the 4 R's, over the next 4 hours, the body will work at replenishing close to 80% of the glycogen stores, provided it gets the right nourishment. And no, it's not complicated: just eating your regular poha / upma / paratha / idli / rice / roti-dal-sabzi or dahi will do the trick.

Your body is keen to make up for the lost glycogen stores and once it does that, its ability to repay the oxygen debt and carry out the repair work of the worn and torn muscle tissues gets easier and quicker. So if you are one of those carb avoiders, then you are gonna lose out on these benefits only to discover that the body is getting insulin insensitive which will tempt you to further reduce carbs which will further weaken the body's glucose uptake and keep you fat. All in all, it's a lose-lose situation.

Also, it will serve you well to remember that Indian meals, or for that matter any native meals where cuisines have evolved over centuries, cannot be broken down into carb, protein or fat like you learnt in school. They are complex mixtures of all these nutrients and are primed to meet the body's nutrient needs by pushing the right nutrient into the blood stream. For example, rice is rich in BCAAs but you learnt to classify it as 'carbohydrate' in school. Now your muscle cells don't read that info you by-hearted in school, so when you eat rice post workout, your body will look up the BCAA structure in them and put them to good use, making glutamine out of it and keeping your immune system from failing. Get it? (And single polished or hand pounded whitish rice is much better than brown rice, read my earlier books for details.)

Chalo, quick recap:

Pre-workout meals	**How it helps**
Gap of 20 minutes or less before workout • Fruit Gap of 60-120 minutes before workout • Homemade breakfast • Homemade lunch • Grilled veg sandwich	• Keeps blood sugars stable during workout • Blunts cortisol response during and post exercise • Allows quicker delivery of glycogen to working muscle group • Minimizes muscle tissue damage
4 R's post workout (within 20, max 45 minutes) • Water • Banana / potato / seasonal fruit • Protein shake (whey) • Vitamins C, E, A, minerals – Se, Zn, Cr	• Makes up for fluid and electrolyte losses during workout • Replenishes glycogen stores and shifts metabolic machinery from catabolic to anabolic • Reduces muscle damage and boosts immune response • Speeds up muscle and systemic recovery • Speeds up elimination of exercise by-products

4 hours post workout Wholesome meals after 1 hour of 4 R's and every 2 hours after that • Poha / upma / idli / dosa / paratha / nachni satva • Dahi / chaas / fruit • Paneer paratha / rice-dal-sabzi / veg pulao-raita / roti-sabzi-dahi	• Maintains increased insulin sensitivity • Sustains the anabolic state • Prevents muscle breakdown and accelerates tissue repair • Allows for maximum glycogen replenishment • Repays O_2 debt and clears out lactic acid • Prevents and repairs neurological damage or damage to motor neurons • Speeds up fat metabolism

The case of whey protein

On my Facebook page and Twitter, the most commonly asked question when it comes to post-workout nutrition is about whey protein. More specifically, these three queries:

1. How to choose a protein shake?
2. But isn't high protein bad for the kidneys?
3. Why can't I have something natural?

There really isn't anything like a poor or high quality protein. All wholesome foods prepared fresh, local and seasonal will provide for good or high quality protein. But the one 'supplement' or 'packaged and processed' food which is worth having, especially if you are a serious weight trainer or weight training for a serious condition like recovery from a fracture, muscular weakness, diabetes, arthritis, heart disease, etc., or just for that leaner, fitter body, is whey protein.

First things first, a supplement means that it will only aid nutrient delivery if diet, exercise and lifestyle are already in place. It isn't an alternative to the real DEAL (diet, exercise and lifestyle), nor is it a drug that causes side effects or addiction or something that the body gets resistant to. A quick example: 'You know, earlier .25 of my sleeping pill would put me to sleep, now even three of those and I am wide awake in the night.' You will never find a weight training enthusiast or an athlete say things like, 'Earlier 20g of protein would help me recover but now it doesn't.'

Whey is a derivative of milk, the white precipitate that curdles to the top while making curd or paneer. The supplement will have it in a concentrated form and flavoured with either chocolate or strawberry and the like to suit people's palates. There are many things that work for whey protein: it's easy digestibility, amino acids (BCAAs as discussed earlier) and bioavailability to name a few. The lactose intolerant can easily consume whey protein too by choosing whey isolate, which is free of lactose.

A protein shake that is easy on your stomach and wallet has the following **per serving (per scoop or per 30 g roughly),** and this is how you should chose your whey protein shake:

Protein: 20-27g

Carbs: 0-3 g

Fat: 0-3 g

It may have many vitamins and minerals added but they are so minute that it is really not very important or critical to look at that. Make sure that the protein mainly comes from the whey, and not other sources. The above ratio of protein to fat to carbs, and the source as whey, pretty much rules out most sugar powders masking themselves as protein supplements on your chemist's shelves.

But isn't high protein bad for the kidneys?

Now that's as much a black and white statement as sugar is bad for health. You've got to dig deeper, understand biochemistry and the body's requirement at any point of time to know if it's 'bad' or 'good' for you. For example, a diabetic who is on the verge of hitting hypoglycaemic coma NEEDS sugar, so sugar is then not just good but very, very good for him.

A person involved in regular exercise has higher requirements of protein than a sedentary individual. If this person already has some disease or a lifestyle disorder, then the protein requirements stand even higher. A protein shake that provides about 25g of protein per serving is not even half a 50 kilo individual's 'daily requirement', so then how is this supposed to be 'bad' for the kidneys? And most of us are heavier than 50 kilos, mind you. Children, geriatric, pregnant and nursing women and adolescents have an even higher requirement of protein.

Btw, everyone needs protein, even a 'kidney patient'. There is absolutely no basis to this fear that protein shakes, especially well-timed protein shakes, can harm the kidneys. It takes much more than 'excess' protein to harm the kidneys, go look at any dialysis ward and let me know if you find even one person there who was regularly weight training or had protein shakes.

The only people who may be prone to kidney disorders are athletes who dope or are on steroids; their kidneys are at a risk and they also typically have protein shakes. But then again, it's not the protein shake that has put them at risk. And if you really want 'most common risk factors' for kidneys, they are dehydration, diabetes and BP, not protein for heaven's sake.

Why can't I have something natural?

If you are asking me this question, you must be a 'social drinker', smoker and occasional doper. Trust me, people with clean lifestyles (ya, I just said yours is not, and no, the what-is-legal-in-Amsterdam argument doesn't stand), who mostly eat at home, work out regularly, are in relationships and professions they like, are never looking for anything 'natural'. Natural, after all, is a state of mind. I mean your toothpaste, your lipstick, your car, your communication via email and video conferences, your e-payments, etc. are all advances and advantages of technology, but protein should be natural as in primitive like meat, eggs, or chal, no problem dal or chana or soya? I mean double standards ki bhi koi limit hoti hai?

The 'natural' chana, sprouts, eggs, chicken, etc. as 'repair' protein in the 4 R's will disturb the blood flow to the working muscle group. And also disturb both the nutrient delivery and waste removal from the damaged muscle tissue. So it will lead to both lack of digestion and assimilation of protein along with delayed glycogen replenishment, and all together it will mean compromised recovery.

What I am saying is, keep it natural everywhere else, in all other meals, and have the protein shake as the R for repair in your 4 R's. It comes from a milk source, and supplements (as against drugs) by regulation or law are not unnatural.

Chapter Summary

Strength training facts

- It's important, in fact critical, to employ the anaerobic energy system in our body
- Strength / weight / resistance training utilizes the anaerobic energy system
- It stimulates the muscle growth and therefore increases the fat -burning capacity of your body
- Strength training improves insulin sensitivity and reduces the risk of developing diabetes
- Strength training using gym equipment ensures you don't get injured and can train at a weight that is lower, at or higher than your body weight
- For a workout to qualify as strength training it has to follow some basic rules:
    - Warm-up should be specific to the main workout
    - Exercise should recruit maximum number of muscle fibres
    - Duration of workout should never exceed 60 minutes
- You can start with as little as 1 hour a week in the gym and gradually build up from there
- A fruit, ideally a banana, is a perfect pre-work out meal
- Post workout, you will need to follow the 4 R's – Rehydrate, Replenish, Recover and Repair
- Whey protein is the most readily digested and natural form of protein that your body can utilize post exercise

Strength training fads

1. Mixing strength training with cardio

Like jumping from one set to another, or exercising body parts in random order — biceps with squats or just after without any rest or kicking high between sets of lat pull down and seated rowing or jumping on tyres and lunging under a bar back-to-back or…

Wait! Wait baba. What are you planning to stimulate today, aerobic or the anaerobic? And even after learning the basic concepts of the energy systems and understanding the time it takes to recover for every energy system, do you really think that 'mixing' is scientific? Most of these 'mixings' attract people who are 'bored' or can't stand 'regular' training, but don't forget that you plateaued or didn't get results with training only because you compromised on the fundamental concepts of exercise science. And don't forget that **compound exercises that employ large muscle groups more than adequately raise your heart rate**; you don't have to jump, skip, run in between sets to do that.

Also, what about the sequence of exercise that you learnt from the basics of strength training plans? Are you being fuel efficient or stimulating muscle growth by just jumping from one 'station' to another? Training or exercising is not the same as exerting or jaan nikal gayee. With any training, no matter how tired it gets you or how much you sweat, if it falters on principles of exercise or the GAS model, you have a person who's exhausted and muscle wasted. And not someone who is adapted and toned, it really is as simple as that.

Similarly, 'circuits' or any other form of training that is a 'mix' or 'fusion' of strength and cardio, or aerobic and anaerobic, is good once in a while, like once in 12 weeks, but not as the whole, or as the basic training program. And if you are super duper fit, then it may interest you as the whole training program for a few weeks, but eventually you have to train the energy systems individually to keep up a training program for years together.

2. Using bands, balls, kettle bells for more fat -burning or as replacement of gym equipment

For starters, remember that the best equipment or machine that you will ever have access to is your body, and to keep that in great shape is the motive, correct? Well then, a lot of the ball, band, suspension ropes category was actually used as rehabilitation equipment to help athletes get back to the gym. Gym equipment, the bars, dumbbells, cable cross rows, or 'machines' running through cams and stuff allows the body to train with maximum safety and efficiency. And only efficient and safe workouts are effective in terms of actually losing weight and making gains in lean body weight.

At other times you may see pictures of super athletes using bands or balls during on-field practice, but remember that they don't 'exclusively' train on this equipment. A lot of their off-season and pre-competition training is in the gym, with machines, which is exactly why they look so lean. So this 'machine free' exercising is at best make-shift, or used as active warm-ups before competition. For example, TRX (suspension ropes) was developed to meet the needs of US marines while they was deployed in 'enemy states' where there was no access to gyms and equipment.

And remember how light, moderate and heavy training is

defined? If you can do more than 15 reps with anything, it's not really stimulating the anaerobic system, so you will lose out on both the systemic and the aesthetic aspects of training this energy system. Also as one more reminder, what matters is how your training is planned in terms of technique, sets, reps and sequence, and not whether you are holding a bar or a band.

Proponents of 'only' body weight, basically all the stuff that is declared as 'machine free' (all working on the principle of more reps, less weight), need to understand EPOC before making tall claims about the fat-burning benefits of this form of exercise. And forget fat-burning, what about the fact that Type 2 and anaerobic pathway is lying unutilized? It is going to lead to muscle breakdown and you will never get that toned look you are aiming for, in fact you will manage to only accelerate ageing and strain your TBLJ.

Strength training FAQs

Q. I have never done any weight training, should I start now?

A. Gosh! Yes, please do. Start with once a week of training and follow through with pre- and post -workout meals. You can make gains in strength at any age and at any stage in life, and any gender, of course.

Q. I have just started weight training, my blood sugar levels are better, my thyroid is better, my jeans are getting loose, everyone's telling me I have lost weight, but I haven't lost a gram, in fact I have GAINED a couple of kilos! :(

A. First things first, change that sad face to a broadly smiling one. Weight training increases fat-free weight, that of your bones and muscles. Obviously that's going to mean some additional grams or kilos to your body mass. Not to forget the fact that as you start storing more muscle glycogen, it adds to body weight too.

Fat is not a dense material, it occupies a large volume on your body, but losing fat weight will mean reduction in body volume much more than reduction in body weight. If your jeans are falling off, you look visibly thinner, and your hormones function better, why get stuck and sad over a number? Move on, come on!

Technically you can lose or gain up to 5 kilos of body weight without gaining or losing a single gram of fat. Body weight is no measure of fatness or fitness. Look at exercise performance instead; it's the sure-shot measure of your body's fat-burning ability (health, fitness and risk of diseases). If you are pushing more weight, feeling more enthusiastic about exercise, looking forward to your routine in the gym, it means you are on track. That's it.

Q: *Gyms didn't exist before a few years, what before that?*

A: Strength training was on even then in our country, with the practice of asanas. But currently 'yoga' has turned into a 'relaxing', 'breathing' or similar form of exercise and we have forgotten that asana practice can be challenging and rejuvenating at the same time (more in the yoga chapter). So yes, if you are one of those types of yoga practitioners, then you wouldn't need to gym. Also years before, people employed their body to carry, lift, move, push many things and therefore didn't need to exclusively train in the gym. Now that we don't carry wood on our heads, pound our rice on our own, make chutneys with stone crushers, we need to gym to keep the muscles alive and active and do so in a safe environment.

Q: *I don't have access to a gym where I live. What can I do?*

A: Start training your anaerobic system through uphill walks, sprints and actively take part in gardening which will require digging, lifting, pounding kind of movements. You will be able to keep the muscles strong and the environment green (please grow local trees and plants). Also practise asanas regularly to help maintain balance between the strength, flexibility and the aerobic and the anaerobic energies.

Q: *But everyone says that once you quit gymming you gain double?*

A: The trick is to not over-commit to the gym (or to any exercise), that way you won't quit. The thing is that gymming brings about maximum changes in the body composition and in all the parameters of fitness, so you start looking good or leaner immediately but quitting means putting an end to the stimuli that caused all these training adaptations. Now the body is intelligent and if you are not going to be needing all this metabolically expensive training adaptations like increased muscle tone, strength, bone density, etc., then the body is better off getting rid of it, the use it or lose it principle is at work. The principle of reversibility also indicates that in the absence of stimuli, the body will let go of its fitness in 2-8 weeks. So take the first 12 weeks slow, put them on the calendar and even if you're training just once a week, be consistent with it, that's your best chance of not quitting. Also in that rare case that you do quit, replace gymming with some equally challenging activity and don't take to lounging.

Q: *Can I sip water between sets? Can I stretch between sets?*

A: Yes you can do both, just stretch the relevant muscle group and don't spend time stretching the entire body between workouts.

Q: *If I am working out in the night then how to plan dinner, protein shake, etc?*

A: The best thing to do if you work out in the night is to have dinner immediately after working out — the dal-rice-sabzi or the sabzi-roti-dal — and have the protein shake after or within an hour post dinner. That way you stay aligned to the 4 R's and keep it real and practical too without pushing dinner too late.

Chapter 4

Cardio

Any cardio activity becomes an exercise only if there is gradual progress in intensity.

'Tell me na, should I run? Bol na meri jaan ... good for my heart and all, haan? GOD! My mother-in-law runs and she had her friends over last night, full 30s se leke 60s-70s ka age group. I was like good, she's got some cool gang ... but oh so boring. Matlab other than running, soreness, injuries, inclines, pasta, carb loading, etc., they talk nothing. NOTHING! I excused myself after dinner was served, I don't think anyone even noticed. After all, I didn't run out of the room, na.'

No, this chapter isn't about how nauseating it can get to be surrounded by running gangs (only the experienced will know that this is not an exaggeration, and God knows they seem to be growing faster than you can say run), it's about running. Ok, no dirty looks for me (I am your favourite author ☺), it's about cardio and knowing how to keep that cardio-respiratory system in shape.

Anyway, before we begin, let me say this:

1. The 'effects', as in the positive effects of cardio, have been exaggerated.
2. Cardio is not the 'go-to' option for fat loss or even weight loss.
3. Nor is it the 'go-to' option for heart health.

4. If you have only 2 days a week to exercise, don't even bother with cardio!

Phew! That's a load off my chest and I feel I am in a sane enough position to now officially start my chapter.

The heart muscle

Speaking of the heart, let's talk about cardiac output. You know how it is these days, nothing is good enough if there is no output or you are as good as your output. Something like that, but with your heart. But before that, some heart-breaking news. You know how you always go to the doctor and learn that the 'normal' heart rate is 72 bpm (beats per minute). Normally we don't want to die by the time we're 66, we want to live longer. So this 72 beats is not 'normal'. Ok, let me explain, I am about to introduce to you the science behind cardio, so that you are not wasting time on the treadmill or breaking your back / knee trying to burn 500kcals.

Let's start with the basic concepts that you absolutely must understand about your heart:

Heart rate (HR) = Number of beats per minute

Stroke volume (SV) = Amount of blood pumped by the heart per beat

And, the cardiac output (Q) = Amount of blood pumped by the heart per minute

So, if I have to relate these three terms, it will be,

Q = HR x SV

Typically, the resting cardiac output (when not physically exercising or under strain) is about 5 litres per minute. Men tend to have about 5.6L per minute and women 4.9L per minute on an average; the difference is because men have larger hearts than women (technically, only). This kind of explains the gap in the running time of elite marathon men and women runners. Anyway, what we need to understand is that right now as you read this (and hopefully you are not reading this while levitating on a cycle or loitering on a treadmill), your heart is pumping close to 5L of blood per minute. Wow! Pata bhi nahi chalta na?

Our heart rate is an indicator of how efficiently we are pumping out this 5L of blood per minute. So if you need 72 contractions (beats per minute) to pump out this 5L, of course your heart is ... ah ... well, average. Now to really have a big heart (not just technically, but really) you must have a much more efficient pumping system. Which means that you should be able to pump those 5L in much fewer contractions.

You know Boris Becker, the great tennis star who won on most surfaces and has multiple records to his name, had a resting heart rate of 32 bpm. So in just 32 beats he would pump out 5L of blood; think about how strong his cardiac muscle was and how high his stroke volume. In fact, any pro-athlete who dominates the scene for over a decade has a really low resting heart rate and this allows him / her to play tirelessly. Our Himalayan sadhus (the real ones) who are supposed to live really long, many will claim meeting someone who was 120 / 150 years old, etc., can lower their heart rate to 3 to 4 beats per minute (it's been documented and proved in labs). So in just 3 or 4 beats they pump out 5L; don't even bother calculating how high their stroke volume is and how big and strong the heart muscle is!

Medical science says that each one of us is born with a certain number of total heartbeats and when we reach that number the heart stops beating. On an average, the human heart has the ability to beat 2.5 billion times. If the average resting heart rate is 72 beats per minute, then we would all die when we're about 66. So if you accept the premise that the heart is born with a certain number of beats, post which is death, but you want to live longer, you must work to lower the resting heart rate to below 72. The way to do that is to exercise; yes, it's as plain and simple as that.

Cardiac output at rest and during exercise

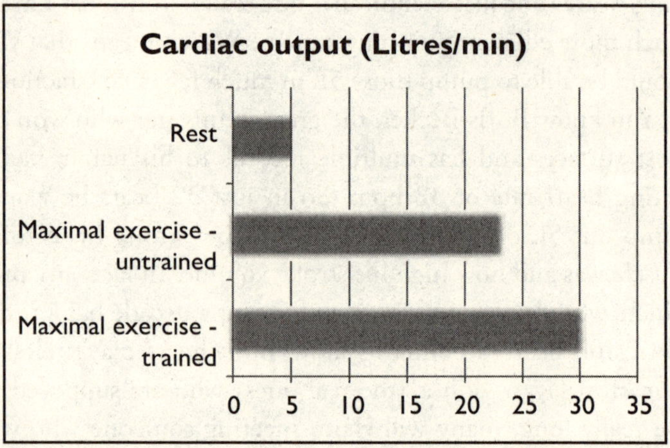

This graph is just to show you how though at rest both trained and untrained or athletes and sedentary have the same cardiac output, athletes can pump much more blood per minute during exercise and that's exactly why they can run faster or perform better than most of us.

Exercise and the heart

One of the many benefits of exercise is that it lowers the resting heart rate (yes, it can do more than fit you into size 6, come on). So let's say that you exercise regularly and as a response to exercise, your cardiac muscle improved and got more efficient with its pumping. So whatever your resting heart was, it now beats one time less per minute than what it used to before you began your exercise program. So you are saving one beat per minute, that is 60 beats per hour, that means 1,440 beats per day, that's 43,200 beats per month and 5,18,400 per year! Now if there was a scheme to save 5,18,400 rupees per year, I am sure you would be on board. But since this is just about health and wellbeing, I am not so sure (ya, ya buying an exercise book doesn't prove your commitment to exercise).

And how does exercise lower heart rate? Remember what we discussed in Chapter 2? About the LV? So, one of the training adaptations to exercise is a more efficient LV — basically a larger chamber and thicker walls with a more efficient capillary network. This means the stroke volume increases, the heart becomes a better pumping machine and the HR decreases. As we also learnt, it's the anaerobic activity that brings about the increase in the capillary network, basically the strength of the heart. And that is one reason cardio for heart health is a misunderstood concept. It is important, but if you really want improvements in heart health, you will need to complement it with anaerobic or strength training.

Technical note — The heart formula

1. Estimate your own maximal heart rate (MHR)
   MHR= 220 – age = _______ bpm
2. Resting Heart Rate (RHR) = _________ bpm (measured first thing in the morning before getting off the bed)
3. Heart Rate Reserve (HRR) = MHR – RHR = _______ bpm

As your RHR decreases, the HRR increases, reflecting an improvement in your heart health. An improved HRR also increases your cardiac output during exercise and therefore your exercise performance or fat burning at any age.

All right, another exercise benefit that is very crucial (no, no, not weight loss, that is just a side effect you see), is the drop in the number of breaths per minute. It's like this, the heart and the lung, your two involuntary organs, work together and make this very beautiful, intriguing and life-sustaining system called the cardio-pulmonary or the cardio-respiratory system. So, as an adaption response, when your resting heart rate goes down, the number of breaths per minute goes down as well.

Slow down

According to the Indian sciences, each one of us is born with a certain number of breaths, and when we exhaust them, we die (not so different from the scientific concept of limited heartbeats). When Bheeshma was on his bed of arrows during the Kurukshetra war, he delayed his death by suspending his breath so that he could finish instructing his nephew Yudhisthir on codes of conduct, dharma and good governance. He delayed his death till he thought that all his duties were done. The story aside, since the heart and lungs work together, when the heart rate drops, breathing rate drops. When the rate of breathing drops, the number of thoughts per minute drops. When the number of thoughts are less, there is less confusion, anger, frustration, and there is more peace, silence and tranquillity. Is this important to you? This more peace, tranquillity, silence part? That way you are not dimaag chabawing at home / office, ha?

Of course, both the lungs and the heart are involuntary, so we have no control over them, unless of course you are Bheeshma ;). However, according to Indian sciences, you can control the involuntary by learning to control your senses. Swami Rama, a great sage from Rishikesh, has proved it beyond doubt in the labs of the West that heart rate and breath can be controlled by sensory control. But most of us have a tough time controlling the voluntary, so involuntary is dur ki baat. So let's focus on that which can be controlled — our muscles are voluntary and they can be trained to listen to us. So run. Arre run. Don't just sit. No? So, voluntary as in they will listen to just you, not to me or anyone else.

So our muscles are voluntary and respond to our 'instructions', and by this very act they become limited, unlike the heart muscle, which is involuntary and can do endless work. Your heart starts beating even before you are born (sometime in the sixth week in the womb) and continues to beat even after death (a few seconds). The muscles, on the other hand, find it tough to contract endlessly and tire out easily.

Imagine I put you on a leg extension machine — how many reps can you really do without getting tired (at any weight). 15? 20? 100? Can you sit there for a lifetime contracting your quads? Nope, a few seconds and you are tired. In fact, some of us have back muscles so weak that we can't even sit upright, we constantly need couches to slouch on, bucket seats to sink into and beds to lie on.

Training the involuntary

Now here's the thing, to strengthen your involuntary muscles (the heart and therefore the cardio-respiratory system), you have to use your voluntary muscles. Just like the heart works with the lungs, the muscles work with the tendons, ligaments, bones and joints (TBLJ), essentially the entire skeletal system. So when you resolve to 'do cardio every day', 'run the marathon' or whatever, what you must remember is that:

- The heart and lungs are infinitely stronger than the TBLJ.
- That without strengthening the skeletal system, you cannot train the cardio-respiratory system.
- That the question, 'Can I just do cardio for weight loss' is a stupid one. Because if you are overweight, your TBLJ will give up way before any fat-burning or improvement of the heart condition can take place.
- And that 'walking is the best exercise' is a lie because, again, your 'best exercise' is limited by the strength of your skeletal system. Or 'if you have diabetes, at least walk' is flawed too because chances are that if you have diabetes / insulin resistance, you are also obese, which means that you have already put more stress on your delicate TBLJ, just by carrying that body weight. Now, if you do decide

to 'walk regularly' with that body weight and frail skeletal system, you will soon need a knee replacement. So your diabetologist will be a happy man / woman — goli chipkane ke saath saath, orthopaedic ka commission bhi. Getting the point?

I don't want to scare you, nor do I want to put you off cardio. I simply want you to understand that it's important for you to have an exercise structure / plan in place. That without planning you will risk an injury and that getting injured and taking bed rest is the exact opposite of getting fit. It's important to use all of the bioenergetics pathways that are available in the human system (Chapter 2). But using the aerobic or the oxidative pathway means 15 minutes or more of exercise or continuous activity, as only then will the body use fat as a substrate (fuel) to allow your muscles to contract (more about this shortly). Doing this meets the primary objective of your commitment to exercise — fat-burning.

While burning fat, your muscles employ the TBLJ to bear your weight and carry you forward (create movement). This causes a strain on your skeletal system, which is very much required, by the way. But without (a) allowing your TBLJ to recover from that strain and (b) actively indulging in stretching and strengthening your TBLJ (rhymes with DDLJ), your 'cardio' / 'aerobics', will take you only that much ahead. And usually this 'that much' is bed rest! Fat burning, full stop!

Periodization and the GAS model

What you require then to continue your commitment to 'fat burning' without phullishestop (foolish stop) is called periodization.

Periodization is an important concept of exercise science (yes, science people, it's a science) and can be defined as an organized approach to training that involves the cycling (or alternating) of different parameters of fitness and energy systems over a period of time.

This periodization is based on the GAS model (the general adaptation syndrome, our biological response to stress) and is divided into three parts:

1. **The alarm stage** — the initial stimuli to the system — choose the right exercise
2. **The resistance stage** — the adaptation to the stimuli — exercise, rest and eat right — increase in fitness, drop in fat percentage
3. **The exhaustion stage** — leading to a poor recovery — not choosing the right exercise, irresponsible eating and inadequate rest leads to a decrease in the systemic response — drop in fitness levels, increase in resting heart rate, increase in body fat percentage

The whole point of periodization is to ensure that the body doesn't reach the exhaustion stage and stays in the resistance stage, adapting, getting younger, fitter, leaner, stronger, faster, sexier. Tudor Bompa is called the baap of sports periodization. He is the one who introduced to the West the concept that training should be cyclical, smart and effective, not exhausting.

Hmm, so now you know why I stated at the very beginning that if you have only 2 days per week to exercise don't even bother with cardio? Dedicate these 2 days to strengthening the TBLJ; without this you will only reach exhaustion of the voluntary system and never come anywhere close to stimulating the cardio-respiratory system. The essential adaptation of improved fat burning, lowered heart rate, breathing and thought rate will be a distant dream. As you have noticed, poor muscular strength or a weak skeletal system often goes hand-in-hand with obesity and poor fitness levels. Working out is the only way to increase the strength of the skeletal system and to lower body fat levels.

Technical note — Bharatnatyam and periodization

Our culture really is so, so fascinating. Just us, as a nation, we have seven classical dances. The aim of our classical dances is sadhana, not fat loss. But to reach a place where sadhana, learning, the very means of spiritual evolution is possible, the physical body must be in great shape. In Bharatnatyam, you study something called adavu (like alphabets, so that you can speak the language of dance). Every adavu is taught to you in a sequence that's been transmitted from generation to generation of nattuvanaars or dance gurus. Now I learn Bharatnatyam, and I was just so intrigued when I discovered the sequence. First came kuditameta, a sequence of dance steps that required me to jump with my heels up but toes down, killed my legs and challenged my brain (came after learning to strike my foot flat and hard on the ground). Boy, my adductors (inner thighs) squealed in pain and I struggled to keep my spine aligned and my hastas decent (alarm stage). Slowly but surely, under my teacher's hawk eye for detail, my body adapted and I learnt to do this with less groaning in the thighs and more control over the fingers, spine, eyes, etc. (resistance stage).

Next came tandutala. Now not just my heels, but also my toes and in fact my feet, my legs, my entire body was mid-air and I was required to keep my spine, hands, eyes, etc. calm, balanced and in mudras (progressive overload). In one action, I whirled around on landing, in another I opened my hands into a petal formation and in a third I struck my right foot. My body and my senses were endlessly challenged. And I wondered if I was doing the right thing for my 'age' (self pity / ego crushing was taking place). My thighs, my hands, my spine, my balance, I felt I was losing everything and I dreaded what would come next. And right then, after tandutala came sarika. It didn't require me to jump, in fact it didn't even require me to sit in aramandi (the half-squat pose that's characteristic of Bharatnatyam). It just required me to step side to side with my feet almost never leaving the ground. Wow! It seemed like a dream post tandutala and it was, for my aching feet, thigh, spine and sore muscles, but now it required me to coordinate the minute muscles of my fingers with my eyes while I leaned forward slightly and stepped side to side.

Sarika relaxed my stimulated skeletal structure; giving it time to adapt and keeping it in the resistance phase without letting it reach the exhaustion stage. At the same time, it shifted the stimuli to another area — hand-to -eye coordination so that a new training concept could be introduced. I was stimulated, relaxed, learning and progressing at the same time.

I wondered aloud to my teacher if her nattuvanaar had ever heard of Bompa or if Bompa had ever looked into our ancient physical training system. Yoga and all our classical dances inherently follow what is now called 'periodization', that's exactly why it didn't burn out or bore students in months / years. The learning stimulated and relaxed at the same time, making students feel that a lifetime wasn't enough to learn. So when you are 'bored' of the gym or aerobics or any other activity, know that it's not lack of consistency from your end, it's the lack of the periodization model in your activity.

So much then for people declaring that 'India doesn't have a culture of fitness'; what we never had is a culture of being frivolous. Our 'fitness culture' employed the physical and sought to go beyond what is visible. Now you do know that the 'training models' discovered sometime in the 1950s and the ones that Olympic winners use were in place in the classical dance and yoga system and they form a part of our collective wisdom bank. Don't equate your unawareness about this with their absence or lack of existence. Please get over yourself (it will help you lose some weight).

Making progress in cardio

If cardio-respiratory progress must be made, then it is important that we learn to use the periodization principle in our cardio workouts. If it's been years and you are walking the same number of rounds in your park, then a) you are not applying the principle of progressive overload and b) by virtue of that, your 'exercise' is a waste of time. When there is no 'alarm' stage or 'new stimuli' there is no reason for the body to adapt or go into resistance stage or to respond by dropping body fat or improving the condition of the heart and lungs. We are goaded to 'walk' with promises like it's good for diabetes, good for weight loss, good for heart, good for God knows what all but we experience that walking hardly ever leads us to actually losing weight or losing our pills. Both stay intact, in fact invariably they climb, the weight in kilos and the pills in dosage.

Now if you must make progress with walking and progressively begin to run and run faster (or swim faster, cycle faster), the TBLJ will have to bear more forces than earlier. Just this point itself is a strong enough argument for you to begin weight training. Without the required strength in your TBLJ, all your cardio efforts land you you-know-where — on the bed, and no, not with a sexy guy / girl but with pain for company.

Strength training, to get better at cardio, will do two things, three actually:

1. Strengthen the TBLJ and the muscles and allow them to bear more forces (as seen earlier, without the required strength in the TBLJ, it will be impossible to train longer or faster in the aerobic zone without risking injuries).
2. Allow you to stimulate the anaerobic pathway that influences and improves your cardio-respiratory fitness and therefore VO_2 max by increasing the lactate threshold (explained below).
3. Train your body to preferentially use fat as a source aerobically and spare glycogen for the anaerobic pathway.

The first, I am sure by now you understand really well. Let's discuss the second and third points.

VO_2 max

This whole 'cardio' is good for you is based on what is called VO_2, your body's ability to extract oxygen from the blood and put it to use in your working muscle. (V – volume, O_2 – oxygen). VO_2 max (maximal volume of oxygen consumed during exercise, measured in ml/kg-min) or **maximal aerobic power is also a measure of your insulin sensitivity and therefore your ability to lose weight, control blood sugar, reduce BP**, etc. — basically your entire metabolic health. Most of us sedentary individuals have a VO_2 max of about 30 ml/kg-min and our man Lance Amstrong has a VO_2 max of about 85 ml/kg-min, so people aukaad mein rehne ka!

It has been observed that the VO_2 max for endurance athletes is the highest as compared to any other sport / activity (and hence the craze for cardio). However, and this is interesting, the top endurance athletes have a VO_2 max which is average or below average for their groups. This points to other factors that must play an important role when it comes to determining cardio-respiratory fitness. The most important training at the lactate threshold.

Lactate threshold

Training at lactate threshold requires runners or cyclists or anyone doing 'cardio' (a term usually used interchangeably with training in the aerobic zone) to move muscles or contract them at a faster speed. This shifts the metabolic gear from aerobic to anaerobic glycolysis, which is a breakdown of the glycogen molecule in the absence of oxygen. Immediately the enzymes, the muscle fibre recruitment, metabolic by-products change too. The muscle goes from using oxidative to unoxidative enzymes, from slow twitch muscle fibres to fast twitch, and there is a huge surge in the metabolic by-product, lactic acid. This point is called the lactic acid threshold (LT) or anaerobic threshold (AT). (And you would want this point to occur as late as possible.) This of course leads to quicker exhaustion of the muscles and turns this 'fast speed' activity into a low duration activity, classical of anaerobic metabolism.

Now though this may not be the speed you run the marathon at or cycle / walk for an hour at, exposure of muscles to the anaerobic zone during the 'cardio' activity will allow you to train at your 'lactate threshold'. This not only recruits Type 2 fibres and prevents their atrophy (breakdown of muscle because of lack of use) but also teaches the body to generate more speed aerobically. **Training at AT/LT, in simple terms running or walking fast periodically in your steady walk / run— will help increase both speed and stamina** by pushing the lactate threshold farther and in effect increase your VO_2 max or your aerobic fitness. If nothing else, it makes cardio more interesting and gets the boredom issue out of the way.

Let's take the example of climbing up stairs. Initially, climbing just 2 floors gets you out of breath and gives rise to a dull ache in your thighs (quads). By the sixth day of you climbing the stairs, the same 2 floors don't get you out of breath or give you any pain in the legs, you feel encouraged to climb up 3 floors. Essentially what you have done is pushed up your lactate threshold and trained your muscles to be more efficient with oxygen. As both aerobic and anaerobic systems improve, over a period of time you look better, leaner and younger.

So the term may sound super fundu, but doing it is very easy. Let's look at its application in running:

	Time	**RPE**
Warm-up run	10 mins	3
Easy run	3 mins	5
Fast run	2 mins	6 - 7
Easy run	3 mins	5
Fast run	2 mins	7

Repeat easy-fast run cycle for 2-3 times.

Over a period of time you will be able to sustain the fast component of the run for longer than 2 minutes, which is an indicator of the fact that you have pushed your LT or in other words, you are getting more efficient with the use of oxygen. You can use the same method if you are walking or cycling, etc. As you progress into your training you will be able to reduce the time spent in the easy phase or the slow component of the workout. The key is to run / walk / cycle at a challenging speed (where you feel like stopping but don't stop), which you can sustain for a few minutes and not run out of breath in a few seconds. This type of training can be undertaken on a day when you have only about 15-20 minutes to work out.

Glycogen sparing — fat burning

Another important way in which strength training helps you make progress in cardio has to do with substrate utilization or the fuel that your body will burn for exercise. Cardio exercises are typically exercises that we perform as 'aerobic' activity, that means we can use glycogen (carb), fat and protein as a fuel. If you perform only cardio / walks / treadmill / cycle and don't weight train, then your body burns a lot more glycogen or carbohydrate before it begins to mobilize fatty acids for exercise metabolism. However the more your body learns and understands that you weight train, which means that you train in your anaerobic zone, meaning that you cannot access any other fuel for training in that zone other than glycogen, the more your body starts 'glycogen sparing' (called as training response or adaptation) by preferentially using fat for aerobic activity and sparing glycogen for anaerobic.

Once this training response takes place, **only then is**

cardio or aerobics a truly fat-burning activity, till that time it's mostly a glycogen-burning activity. And no wonder then that you are not seeing the results you want to, in spite of investing time in 'brisk walking daily'.

Technical note — Second wind

Chemically, the carbohydrate and fat molecule consists of carbon, hydrogen and oxygen atoms. The difference lies in the fact that carbohydrate is richer in oxygen and fat is poorer. So in the initial stages of cardio, when your body has just increased its breathing rate and started providing oxygen to the working muscle, the body will burn carb, and over a period of time, switch to burning fat. This is also another reason why a nice warm-up is required so that even metabolically your body will switch effortlessly from burning carbs to burning fat. I am sure you have noticed this: you begin running, let's say, and the first 10 to 15 minutes really seem difficult and you hate yourself for being so fat / unfit / out of shape, etc. Suddenly, like something has changed, like a fresh lease of life, the doubts disappear, the breathing evens out, the legs seem to move in an automatic rhythm and the effort level drops. If you were able to go deep within your body, you would notice that the ATP is now coming out of fat versus carbs, and since fat is an unlimited source you will feel that you can now go on forever. Technically, there's a term for this feeling, it's called the second wind.

Cardio in practice — from knowing to doing

How should you start with your cardio workout? Which cardio activities should you chose? How should you ensure your cardio workout stays in the resistance stage, that it follows the principle of progressive overload and that it fits into your limited exercise schedule? Let's learn.

1. The FITT formula
2. The training diary
3. Application to walking and swimming
4. Running and marathon training

1. The FITT formula

I am going to introduce you to a very effective training tool, it's called the FITT formula — frequency, intensity, time and type of exercise. This formula has the principle of periodization built into it, **it forces you to rotate the time, intensity and type of exercise and ensures that you don't burn out or get exhausted because of exercise.** In effect, it ensures that you don't mouth dialogues like, 'Har roz chalta hoo, but BP niche nahi aaya', or 'All the cardio on earth and my triglycerides are shooting through the roof', or 'I am going to quit, saala full time waste, I would rather sleep 20 minutes extra and read all the gossip in *Mumbai Mirror*'.

So if we apply this formula to cardio, and take a very practical scenario, it will be like this:

Frequency — twice a week
Intensity — one day hard, one day easy
Time — one day 20 minutes, and one day 40 minutes
Type – cardio (walk or run or cycle or swim, etc.)

Frequency and time — For most of us, frequency and time will be easy to determine, and as you read the chapter and the book you will figure out how to plan your workout week.

We are going with 2 days, one for 20 minutes and one for 40 minutes, as the most practical scenario. (Note that this is in addition to the days / time spent doing anaerobic / strength training or yoga, etc.)

Intensity — When the intensity is high, reduce the time and when the intensity is low increase the time. An easy and a hard day essentially means that both aerobic and anaerobic pathways will get utilized. I am sure you know how to determine hard and easy: no, not by measuring your heart rate, but by using the RPE scale (Chapter 2 again). On the easy day stay at '5' and for the hard day stay at '7'.

Type – This is where you will need to figure what works best in your case. Let's look at this in detail.

Choice of cardio type

On days you are doing high intensity, choose a surface that is kind to your TBLJ — so walk / jog on grass, sand, or better still, swim or cycle. You can choose swimming and cycling on the easy days of 40 minutes too, the only reason why I am not forcing you to stick to swimming and cycling on the light days too is because it's easier for me to get you to do 'inconvenient' tasks for a shorter duration. Apart from convenience, the two factors that will help you choose the type of cardio activity on hard days are:

1. How time-consuming the activity is: Going to the pool or bringing the cycle down a lift or transporting it to places where you can finally cycle is time-consuming. And since most of us lead busy lives and can barely spare about an hour for 'low-priority' activities like exercise, it just makes sense na, to keep time-consuming activities as short bursts

of high-intensity exercises. This allows you to keep the TBLJ safe too.

2. The post-workout meal: The medium in which you train influences your appetite. Train in water (swimming) and you will feel super hungry post exercise, train on land (walk or run) and you almost feel like throwing up at the sight of food. Now eating is going to take time too, so to build a sustainable exercise program that doesn't unduly stress you out about your schedule, opt for water exercises when you are planning to up the intensity. Higher intensity, or going towards 7 or 8 on the RPE scale, means working out at a higher exercise heart rate. This means faster and more intense movements in the skeletal system, so it's best done in the natural shock absorption system that water provides. And then because it's just 20 minutes, you have enough time to eat (or hog) as compared to when you do a lighter workout of 40 minutes and use land as a surface or training medium, then you are not as hungry so you don't need too much time to finish your post-workout meal.

So swimming and walking / running on soft surfaces (sand, grass, mud) are good options for high-intensity cardio days, but let's look at some alternatives too:

a) *No access to pool and / or don't like swimming*

Now of course all of us are not going to have a pool to go to or may not even know how to swim. So if you have access to a pool and don't know how to swim, learn, and if you truly don't have access to a pool, cycle. If you are completely out of shape, choose a stationary bike, and over a period of time learn to cycle on roads. Cycling on roads requires you to be more alert in terms of traffic and other movement, which in turn recruits more nerves per unit muscle fibre and leads to better neuro-muscular co-ordination.

b) ***Don't want to either cycle or swim***

And if you are absolutely stuck up and just won't cycle or swim, then begin with buying good shoes for your walking activities. In the beginning, i.e., the first couple of months, you will have to 'retire' your workout shoes quickly as your muscular and TBLJ weakness will wear out its shock absorption abilities at a rather fast speed. So after 2 months, max 3, shift them to 'my shoes to wear with jeans' instead of my shoes to walk. As you gain more strength in your musculo-skeletal system and drop fat mass, you may use the same pair of shoes for about 6 months, but retire they must, and in a country like ours, you can even just donate them and there will be many takers for your charity. Of course all this is if you actually log in cardio sessions twice a week from date of purchase, and have not just bought the shoes, kept them in the cupboard and then, 'Oh, 2 months are over so let me buy new ones', get it?

c) ***Everything inside the gym only***

Now it is absolutely possible that you may not swim, walk or cycle outdoors and are a complete gym junkie. In that case you can increase intensity (or strain on the musculo-skeletal system) in the following order — cycling, elliptical, treadmill. Cycling, as we all know, does not require the body to carry its own weight. The elliptical or cross-trainer simulates a running-like motion but requires you to keep your foot in touch with the pedal at all times, thus reducing the stresses and strains that go through the weight-bearing joints. The treadmill, with its moving belt, simulates a walking or running motion and allows free movement for your feet, so it will put more strain on the TBLJ than the elliptical or the cycle. So keep the treadmill for the easy or low-intensity days. But then comes the other problem, most gyms have a 20-minute-only policy for treadmills. So for your long-duration, low-intensity days, start with the treadmill and then go on to the elliptical or cycle; basically as the joints get more tired, take them to a machine that will provide them some relief and ensure that the voluntary system, the musculo-skeletal structure, can continue stimulating the cardio-pulmonary system without harming itself or going through irreparable damage.

d) *Recovering from injury*

Now, if you are one of those cry babies who are recovering from back / knee / ankle injury and is in a 'my doctor says that I need to work out but I just can't do cardio right now' situation, here's what you can do — row. Rowing machines in the gym put your lower body in a fixed, steady state and give your upper body, more specifically your back, shoulders and arms, a good cardio workout.

2. The training diary — count what matters

Just logging in 2 days a week won't bring you fat loss, protect your joints and make your cardio-pulmonary system more efficient — counting your effort will. Ever wondered why all we do is count results, spending so much time and resources doing that, when all that matters is effort? And no, desperation doesn't count as effort, so just because you are more desperate to lose weight it is not going to automatically or magically lead you to a lower body weight. Anyway, there is an easy method to count what you do, it's called the training diary or exercise log / tracker. To understand how to read it and how to interpret what you read, let's look at an example.

Example of a training diary for cardio:

Exercise	Surface	Resistance	Time	Distance	RPE	Enjoyment	Date
Cycling	Road	Nil	20 mins	5	6	7	2/5/13
Walking	Grass	-	40 mins	3	4	9	5/5/13
Elliptical	Gym	2	20 mins	2.7	7	5	8/5/13
Swim	Water	Shallow	20 mins	4 laps	Dead	10	12/5/13
Rowing	Gym	1	10 mins	Not sure	6	3	15/5/13

The most important columns are the RPE and enjoyment. Now you can see from the enjoyment rating — where 1 is the least and 10 is 'I am having too much fun' and 5 is 'Ok, not bad' — that this person seems to enjoy walking on grass and swimming the most. Enjoys cycling on the roads too, but rates the indoor cardio activities a bit low. Now **the minute boredom sets in, consistency with exercise comes under a serious threat.** When you enjoy what you do, you are likely to do it even when you are hard-pressed for time, had a late night or have an early morning meeting / flight to catch. Life is invariably dealing with one of these or other challenges and when faced with a choice of boring exercise and saving time or simply sleeping five minutes more, our chances of choosing the latter are, you know how high.

It's important that we must be stimulated by exercise itself and not by its promise to bring us better health. It's like a lifelong relationship where you must be stimulated by your partner and not the stability or security a marriage may provide. When in love you are ready to cross the Sea Link going from south Mumbai all the way to Juhu to pick / drop your loved one. When you lose interest in the relationship, the same distance becomes ALL THE WAY TO JUHU!! Sea Link is bloody 60 bucks one way and what not! Basically, jahan dil nahi lagta wahan waqt nahi guzarta.

So coming back to the point, date / explore several forms of cardio to figure dil dhak dhak kiske saath karta hai. And once you are driven by love and passion for exercise, then every excuse will pale in the face of the exhilaration that it will bring.

Technical note — The stages / groups of cardio

World-over, fitness bodies — like the ACSM — divide cardio-respiratory exercises into three distinct stages, based on the wear and tear it puts the body through and the skill requirements. Obviously, as you get fitter, you can both bear and recover faster from wear and tear as compared to when you are unfit or just starting out.

Stage 1 or Group 1: Walking, jogging, elliptical, cycling (on a stationary bike), climbing stairs, rowing (on the stationary rowing machine)

Stage 2 or Group 2: Running, aerobic dance classes, group cardio classes, skipping rope, cycling (on a real bike), swimming, skating, skiing, etc.

Stage 3 or Group 3: Racquet sports, volleyball, basketball, etc.

However, it's important to understand that this is a very generalized grouping and points much more towards the skill and fitness that every activity requires and is not necessarily a step-by-step guide as to how you must progress with your cardio training (although it can be used as one). Many children, adolescents and teenagers may be actively indulging in Group 3 and 2 activities, but that doesn't mean that they have to be first taught how to do activities in Group 1. They may in fact find them extremely boring as their sports skills and VO_2 is already much higher than the stimuli that Group 1 activities may provide.

---

3. Planning your cardio workout — Examples of walking and swimming

To progressively overload on cardio means working on improving one of the three parameters of FITT — Frequency, Intensity or Time — coz 'Type' is constant and stands for cardio. Given most of our schedules, it's tough for us to add another day and increase frequency or make an additional investment of 20 minutes to our (threatening to fall apart anytime) existing workout routine. Also, purely in terms of recovery, adding another day of cardio may not be a great thing for the TBLJ, or even making them undergo the stress of carrying forward our body weight for another 20 minutes may be more foolish than prudent.

So if you are shaana, then you will increase intensity, which means that eventually you will move to running from walking. And no, a 'brisk walk' doesn't count. I mean, for how many years or months do you think that this 'I do brisk walking' is gonna stimulate the system? Max, and this is if you are beginning at exceptionally poor fitness levels (in which case, you shouldn't walk and khao daya on your TBLJ), 12 weeks. Sustained stimuli will bring changes in 12 weeks; beyond that, if the stimulus doesn't increase / change, there will be deterioration. Anyway, there has to be an overload, meaning that the muscles should encounter forces more than what they are accustomed to, if they are to hypertrophy and with them both the musculo-skeletal and the involuntary system (heart, lungs) hypertrophies.

Let's go back to the training diary in the example above. We can see that walking and swimming are high on love, so applying our FITT formula, and progressively increasing the intensity, we can plan a workout using just grass or water as a surface. Here is how:

a) Walking — group 1 cardio activity

As he progressed with his routine, his weekly schedule for walking looked like this:

Week 1

Exercise	Surface	Resistance	Time	Distance	RPE	Enjoyment
Walk	Grass	-	40 mins	3 rounds around the park	4	9
Walk–run	Grass	10 meter jog every 5 mins	20 mins	Approx 1.5 rounds	8	8

Week 4

Walk	Grass	-	40 mins	3.2 rounds	5	10 (covered more ground in same time)
Walk–run	Grass	10 meter jog every 4 min	20 mins	Almost 2 rounds	8	8.5 (good fun)

Eventually, this is what it looked like:

Week 12

Exercise	Surface	Resistance	Time	Distance	RPE	Enjoyment
Walk	Grass	Doing some slopes in between	40 mins	4.5 rounds	5	9 (made some super friends)
Walk–run	Grass	Not needing to walk now	20 mins	Almost 3 rounds	8	10 (fab run)

A detailed description of how exactly to progress week by week in your walking is given in Chapter 6 under the principles of exercising right.

So if you apply the FITT formula right, your hard and fast days of 20 minutes will soon lead you to progress from walking to jogging and eventually running. This is when the load on your weight-bearing joints may just shoot up and if cardio is not accompanied by strength training and stretching, then it will lead to issues in the TBLJ. We will discuss more about running shortly, but let's first look at another cardio activity — swimming.

b) Swimming – group 2 cardio activity

Applying FITT to swimming, the progress looked like this:

Week 1

Exercise	Surface	Resistance	Time	Distance	RPE	Enjoyment
Swim	Water	-	20 mins	5 laps with floating / backstroke in between	8	9
Swim	Water	-	40 mins	Lost track of laps but swam continuously with only 5-6 breaks of 2 mins max	6	10 (gossiped with Neha all along)

Week 12

Swim	Water	-	20 mins	8 laps	8	9
Swim	Water	-	40 mins	4 breaks of 2 mins	7	9

Basically, what you need to know is that applying the high / low formula (FITT) and using different bio-energetic pathways is easy by varying the intensity and keeping the activity or surface constant. The charts also depict progress or training adaptation where you can see that RPE remains near constant even with increased stimuli or effort in exercise. You can use the training diary as above to track your efforts and progress with exercise so that it remains meaningful and joyful.

Training as a hobby

The two people who often take to 'training' others as their 'hobby' are doctors and 'homemakers'. Now I am sure you understand that training is a big science by itself, and it needs to be pursued and practised with the seriousness of studying the laws of dynamics or whatever. Teaching people or being responsible for planning workouts for human beings will mean proficiency in at least the basics of kinesiology, physiology, exercise science, biomechanics, ergonomics, nutrition, motivation, communication, behaviour science, etc. And being a housewife or a doctor offers no advantage in being able to learn these subjects or in your ability to apply the learnings to other human beings. The big reason why these two people choose to pursue this hobby of 'training' is because anything associated with weight loss is a good money-making proposition. So if you must learn or get trained under the housewife / doctor, ensure that they have the required training to do so and have the confidence to call this their calling and career and not time pass or hobby. And yes, having a fit / thin body yourself or completing some random marathon is no qualification to start telling people what to do about their fitness or lack of it. Thinness is not fitness.

4. Running and marathon training

As a child you run all the time: run to open the door, run to school, up and down the stairs, just about everywhere, in fact some schools very foolishly punish students who are found 'running in the corridor'. Believe it or not, you were once very much at a mitochondrial age where running all the time came naturally to you, and walking seemed like a punishment. But now here you are, not as light on your feet as you used to be, not because you gained weight but because you lost muscle strength, mostly from your hips, lower back and inner thighs.

Running may seem just like walking that has gone hyper but it really is very different. If you were to do a GAIT analysis, i.e. study of the way your foot strikes and leaves the ground, you would notice dramatic differences between walking and running. In fact, every person's GAIT is unique in nature, almost like your fingerprints. A blind person can figure out who has come based on the way the foot strikes the ground, so even without being able to see, they would know it's the paternal grandmom or the maternal, the neighbour or the friend from class. The film industry will tell you that no one walks like Sanju baba, not even Salman, and that they loved the way Mamta Kulkarni walked. Poets have described the gait of women very romantically as nagin jaisi chaal, to describe the sway of the hip. The point is, if the strength in the hip reduces dramatically, and it can, simply out of disuse (because you sit so much), then the nagin will spiral out of control and it will look anything but romantic or appealing. You will find many such women and men walking around in India's parks. In fact, I propose that there should be a special mobile unit which goes around all the joggers' parks, picking up these men and women and dropping them off at the nearest Iyengar yoga class or weight training studio.

So when you walk, at any point of time, one foot remains in full contact with the ground, and the lower back, hip, knee and ankle (your weight-bearing joints) have to support your bodyweight. Now as you start running, you have something called as the 'non-contact phase', when both your feet are mid-air. This is often the favourite of most photo journalists and you will see pictures of your city's marathon with the Kenyan runners mid-air either at the start or at the finish.

Running is characterized by this phase where both feet are off the ground and then, even as one foot lands, the other one is off the ground. Because of the forces (gravity) and velocity involved, you **will land with 2 to 3 times as much weight on your landing leg as compared to walking**. And you don't stop but work at moving that weight forward by going into another non-contact phase. Imagine what happens to the weight-bearing joints They go through immense forces and the muscles go through eccentric contraction, i.e. they lengthen as they contract under gravity. **Eccentric contraction, lengthening during muscle contraction, is also the phase where most injuries take place.** It's always on landing that people get hurt, they are never hurt mid-air or on take-off.

This doesn't mean you should be scared of running; we have already discussed that if your walking is not progressing to running, it's not an exercise anymore and doesn't give you any benefits associated with exercise, in fact it will only harm you. What it means is that you need to be smart about running, plan it properly, include strength training as an essential component, train at lactate threshold, strengthen your core, stretch your muscles and be willing to take the disciplined approach.

Marathon-ing

We can't talk about running and not talk about the latest and greatest in thing — MARATHON! Mumbai mein din mein, Bangalore mein raat ko, Ladakh mein snow pe, Rajasthan mein sand pe, not to forget the London, Boston, Paris marathons. You can't be living in a metro and have not come across a group of runners, with pride and pain on their faces, running on the roads as they train for the marathon.

What is it about marathons that hook the non-athletes (mostly the 40 and above)? Plenty! But because it's beyond the scope of this book, I'll only talk about what's most obvious (with a bit of bitching).

1. It's the only 'sport' on earth that allows you to tread on the same ground as the elite athlete. The guy who comes first and you who come last (chal na, almost last, ok chalo, middle) all get to run on the same road, same route. And if you are amongst the biggies in the city, or belong to the company who is sponsoring the run, or to one of the big running clubs in the city, then you even get to stand right behind these heroes. Yes, heroes. Athletes, men and women, are heroes. They run the marathon in little over 2 hours and the 21 km in a little over 1 hour. You run the marathon in a little under 5 hours mar mar ke, and 21 km under 2½ hours mar mar ke (and you know I am not exaggerating here).

2. Also, when the population is generally lazy, you are treated like a role model, someone who gets a standing ovation in office, a mention by the boss at the sales meet, etc., simply because you participated and completed the run! Timing ko maro goli and you maro big dialogues like, 'I didn't know I had it in me to run the marathon', 'Now I know if you

put your mind to it, nothing is impossible', etc. Boss, wait for a second, any other sport and you wouldn't even get a chance to watch it, so how about humility for a second, ha? And if you complete the run in just double the time of the elite athlete, less than 4 hours for 42 km and sub 2 for 21 km, phir toh boss, you are like, like, I don't even know the right word for it. Matlab! The whole damn world doesn't even know what an achievement that is! Now try running 100m in 20 seconds (double of Bolt) and you will be able to run, but there will be no such speeches, mentions, chance to stand somewhere behind him or let your lotus feet touch his track. But marathons allow you that privilege.

3. If you meet 10 marathon runners (and you will always meet more, because they move around in packs) and ask them if they were into sports earlier like in school and stuff, they will proudly say — NO! Never (most of them are scholar types). Ok, chalo at least nine of them won't be into anything, there may be the odd one who's actually been sporty in the past. And there is a reason for that. Marathon or running long distance involves the Type 1 or the oxidative muscle tissue. The sporty ones are the ones with dominant Type 2 muscle tissue, so they never really 'feel' like a long run. But the way the running gangs are growing, people who have played hockey, kho-kho, basketball, football, etc. in school are feeling, 'are we really sporty enough if we don't run the marathon?' To them I want to say yes, yes, you are, my sweety. With age, the Type 2 muscle tissue wears out at a faster rate, so go back to the field, but back to your game, not just to long-distance running.

4. Moreover the nature of marathon running means that participation itself is everything; it's about showing up at the start line; when you finish is not really all that important. Suits the non-sporty types perfectly well, they are anyway unused to physically pushing themselves. They are good at analysis. So you will find these runners with more gadgets than someone who is about to propel a rocket into space. They will 'measure' and then analyze everything — their start time, stride efficiency, whether they are running at 6kmph or under and 'predict' their finish time. That's their game, numbers. Will they do anything about the numbers for the next run? Change the way they approached training for the run? Get to the gym and improve their core? Understand that stretching or upper body strength is crucial for 'good timing'. Nope! They train exactly the same way they trained earlier; they just switch to more expensive shoes, gadgets and take part in philosophical discussions about running.

Anyway, to cut a long story short, just because you have the privilege and money (the shoes and gadgets cost a bomb) to run you shouldn't do so just to fit in. I mean, be kind to your TBLJ, train them, strengthen them, care about your VO_2 and know that timing should get less and less every year, not more and more. Also, that getting injured shouldn't be 'normal'. You are, after all, what is called as the recreational athlete. If you run the full marathon sub 2.5 hours and have some knee issue, that's fine, but finishing in 5 or 4 hours and having joints that hurt is not ok. Please approach your training in a scientific manner. Also please,

please don't go to office and say to the 20- and 30-year-olds things like, 'Come on man, you should run the marathon', or worse, 'You youngsters should be staying fit, learn from us', etc. Please, it's not motivating, it's desperate. A desperate attempt to tell the young testos and estos that you have 'arrived'; if you really have, look it, man. Lose that paunch. Look like a runner. Think Milind Soman!

Runner 'bad' looks

And really, I never thought this day would come in my lifetime (or at least so soon), when someone would actually say to me, 'But I don't want to look like a runner.' I am pre-programmed to hear, 'But I don't want to look like a body builder', so I almost started rattling off, 'Don't worry, it is quite difficult to get that look blah blah...', and then suddenly I had to stop myself in my tracks.

It is quite easy to get that wasted muscle and high body fat look especially if you are one of those people who run in double or more of the elite timing. And even if you are not high on body fat, to get that wasted muscle look is quite easy, there are basically three main reasons for that:

1. Lack of training in the anaerobic zone and at lactate threshold (which utilizes and recruits the Type 2 muscles).
2. Lack of strength training to maintain strength in the TBLJ and muscle, and lower body fat.
3. Lack of proper meal planning, especially around the big runs.

Sadly, most of our runners, even the ones who run 5 to 7 days a week regularly, don't look fit, sharp, lean and young, and ironically most of them sport a paunch and have a haggard look about them. It's ok to look haggard post a run, and that too only for a little while, but not otherwise. This, 'I don't want to look like a runner', describes an over-trained runner (or cardio enthusiast) basically because of the three things overlooked or entirely absent from the workout plan.

If running is your thing, you must run and train, but realize that there is much more to marathon training than joining a group and talking about high-funda stuff. In fact, there is so much that it deserves a book by itself (and perhaps I will write one soon). Till then, I am sharing with you a training plan for the half marathon (21 km) from one of our previous Mumbai marathon trainings, after applying the FITT formula and keeping into account all that we have learned about exercise science.

The 14-week training plan for 21 km (half-marathon)

Week	Monday	Tuesday	Wednesday	Thursday	Friday	Saturday	Sunday
1	-	-	CSB / 1.3K	-	-	CSB / 2.0K	LR / 4K
2	CT	ST	SR / 2.0K	Rest	ER / 3.0k	CSB	LR / 6K
3	Rest	ST	SR / 3K	ER / 3k	ST	CSB / 1K	LR / 7K
4	CT	LT / 2K	LR / 6K	Rest	CSB / 2k	ST	Rest
5	ER / 3K	CT / 30 min	SR / 3K	LT / 3K	ST	CSB	LR / 7-9K
6	Rest	CT / 40 min	SR / 4K	ER / 6K	ST	CSB / 3K	LR / 8-10K
7	Rest	CT	LT / 4K	ER / 6K	ST	CSB / 2k	LR / 9 -11K
8	ER / 3-5K	ST	SR / 3K	LT / 6 -8 k	CT / 30mins	CSB	LR / 12 K

9	Rest	CT	LT / 4K	ER / 6-8K	ST	CSB	LR / 14-16K
10	Rest	CT / 50 min	SR / 4K	ER / 7-9K	ST	CSB / 2K	LR / 16-18K
11	Rest	CT / 20 min	SR / 4K	ER / 10K	ST	CSB	LR / 16K
12	Rest	CT / 20 min	SR / 4K	ER / 8-10K	LT / 6K	CSB / 2k	LR / 16-18K
13	Rest	CT / 30 min	SR 2.5K	ER / 5K	ST	CSB	LR / 10-12K
14	Rest	CT / 40 min	SR / 3-5K	ER / 2 K	LT / 20 min	CSB	D-day / 21K

CSB	Core strength and balance
LR	Long run
CT	Cross training (cycling, swimming, etc)
ST	Strength training in the gym
SR	Steady pace run (road running)
ER	Easy run (on a soft surface)
LT	Lactate threshold

Recreational sports

If you look at the grouping earlier in the chapter you will see that the Group 3 cardio activities include most racquet sports, basketball, volleyball, etc. So these fitness bodies recognize that racquet sports place more wear and tear on your body than most other forms of cardio. These are also the sports that more and more people are playing for recreation. And most of them are again in their 40s.

No, I have nothing against the age group, my body will get to the number 40 too, this isn't about the age, it's about the attitude and lifestyle. So a lot of people in their 40s have last played a game of tennis in school or at that holiday in Ooty during college internship or as a part of the production versus sales team match at their first job. Cut to present, they are at a good place in their life, gaadi, bungla, living in one of those huge complexes which separate the rich from the poor and gives these 40-year-olds unconditional access to the tennis, squash, badminton courts along with gym and swimming pool facilities.

Guess what activity my 40-year-old will try first? The tennis / squash / badminton, of course! It's aspirational not in terms of fitness but only in terms of status; I mean, only the rich in our country have access to these things, right? And then what, the oft-repeated story — arre 3 days I played squash, mera ankle sprain ho gaya; squash is very injury prone. Or replace squash with tennis / badminton / basketball / volleyball and they are all 'injury prone'. And that, my little Miss Muffetts and Clueless Bunties, is because of the lack of strength in the TBLJ, the poor VO_2 and the rusty skill that make you prone to injuries, not the game. You just continue to sit around more, longer than what you have, and even travelling in the car, picking up the suitcase from the belt, taking an international flight will become 'injury prone' or 'restricted'. You don't use your muscles, you lose them, buddy.

But then all is not lost, that one game you played sometime somewhere, many years ago, will bless your muscles with memory. The next time you approach the game with somewhat similar body composition or strength in the muscles, your muscles will bless you by re-igniting that memory of the skill, VO_2 max and the other jargon that you may have learnt by now. You can get to that body composition by being patient with your body and staying consistent with your Group 1 cardio along with weight training activities for about 12 weeks. (To learn how, check 'The player' workout analysis in Chapter 6.)

Time time ki baat hai jaani :). Memory is a funny thing, it's nowhere and everywhere. Play the way you used to, and you will even start thinking about the girl who sat on the first bench and looked at you coyly when you smashed the opponent's shuttle. You hadn't thought about her in ages and you hadn't hit that shuttle with so much power in ages, one comes back so does the other. Am I scaring you now? Oh come on, just the memory comes back not getting caught passing chits to her ;).

So, in short, you do anything that is not a challenge to your system and it gets too boring to continue or sustain that activity. You do anything that's way higher than your fitness levels and it gets challenging to sustain activities, again because of the risk of injuries. With everything in life, including fitness, walk the 'madhayama marg', the golden path according to the Buddha, one that challenges but not exhausts.

Meal planning for cardio

If protein is the buzzword for weight training then it is carbs for cardio. Regular gymmers (yeah, I just invented that word inspired by the Mumbaiya 'batter' for batsman ;) seem to unanimously agree that protein is essential for lifting weights, cutting fat mass and rippling muscles. The cardio crowd however seems confused, there's either a no carb before workout diktat or swallowing of carb gels and 'energy' drinks during workouts. So let's try and remove the veil of confusion from fuel for cardio.

Fuel for Cardio

Our body breaks down the food we eat to produce energy, but it's not a straightforward conversion. This is how it happens (I know you were traumatized by chemistry so will keep it short): Carbs, fats and proteins from food get converted to a chemical called 'Acetyl – Coenzyme A' and then this Acetyl–CoA after all the electron transport jazz produces ATP (the whole process is called Krebs cycle). The human body is a democratic institution and believes in the uniform civil code — carb, fat or protein, everything to Acetyl–CoA and eventually to ATP. Samjha kya? Just because you belong to the 'majority' who rants weight loss, weight loss, your body will not let go or flex its rules and burn only fat for you.

But we have learnt (in the strength training chapter) that the body can be trained to spare glycogen and instead use fat as fuel for cardio if you are regular with anaerobic exercise that exclusively relies on glycogen as a source. Using your anaerobic pathway, with strength training, sprints, fast jogs interspersed with your walks, is the way to teach your body that. But what else can you do to increase fat burning during cardio exercises? Eat more fat. Yes, you read that right. And here is why.

Eat fat to burn fat

Our body typically stores fat as triglycerides in both the fat cells (or the adipose tissue) and in the skeletal muscle cell. When the body employs the aerobic pathway then it breaks down triglycerides from the adipose tissue (also called as adipocytes) into free fatty acids and transports it via the blood to the working muscle tissue.

Now consumption of dietary fat (natural, unprocessed — ghee, makhan, coconut, the tadkas in your sabzis, etc.) also leads to an increase in the free fatty acids (FFA) in the blood stream. Also because of certain mechanisms, FFA in the blood due to dietary fat seems to encourage both the breakdown of stored triglyceride in the fat cells into FFA and its utilization by the working muscle tissue. Together this process leads to more utilization of fat as a fuel source and sparing of glycogen. The **sparing of glycogen and better utilization of fat leads to better exercise performance and less fatigue in the working muscle tissue.** Yes, yes, obviously more fat burning and therefore reduction of body weight and volume due to loss of fat mass also.

Why am I telling you all this? So that you don't avoid fat in your diet. Remember that ghee and coconut, due to the structure of the carbon atom chains in them, are specially primed to increase workout performance and calorie burning. The supplement stores in New York City are packing their shelves with 'performance enhancing ergogenic aids' — basically, clarified butter and virgin coconut oil. Our diets are naturally rich in both, so please don't fall prey to fads, eat your regional cuisines and don't do soup salad or only fruit or oats upma for dinner. Your grandma was right, and now there is research to prove it — muscle triglyceride stores and their utilization plus uptake of FFA from the blood stream to provide energy / stamina is greater when 'divine' fats like ghee and coconut are on your thali.

But when to consume the fat? Just before an exercise session? No, the night before, if you work out in the morning. And if you work out in the evening, then the lunch should be wholesome and ghee on your rotis is a must.

Carbs are important too

But the body learns to preferentially use fat only after you are consistent with training, and even then carbs are the fuel to kick-start the exercise. But when you are beginning or have not yet reached a particular fitness level, the demands on your glycogen stores are much higher

Now as you start exercising, the muscle glycogen levels start depleting and the muscles begin experiencing fatigue. So you may really want to walk for 10 minutes more, or run a little faster, but the muscles will not be able to keep up with the demand. This happens mainly because of two reasons: the blood sugars drop leading to hypoglycaemia, and dehydration sets in. Also, let's not forget that the brain almost exclusively operates on glucose, so with hypoglycaemia, even the brain starts to work against your will to exercise, giving rise to thoughts like — Chal na, let's work out tomorrow / I will never be able to climb this slope / Forget it, this bitch looks so much slimmer than me / Ouch, ouch let me move more slowly / Let me just stop, sit in a rickshaw and go home, etc. Basically it prevents you from exercising to prevent larger issues that may come up just because of lack of glucose to the brain. In short, you never reach the stage in your exercise where your body is now burning fat

Accidents and hypoglycaemia

Empty stomach cardio or just coffee and cardio are especially lethal for people who run, cycle on roads or drive to gyms. After overnight fasting (sleeping), your body has lost almost 80% of its glycogen stores. So when you wake up and eat nothing or just maaro a coffee, your body doesn't magically burn fat, but burns whatever carbs are left and then turns to the precious muscle tissue instead, and you stay fat. Well, there's something worse than that, and that's going out in a low-carb, and therefore low blood sugar state, which reduces glucose availability to your brain. Now you must remember that living in India means that pedestrians, runners, cyclists are second-class citizens, so expect cars to not slow down for you, and if you look sexy enough then for cars to slow down and come dangerously close to you simply to check you out. Or if you live in Mumbai, then the rickshaw driver to slow down close to you and say something very flattering, like 'kya saix' and the likes. Now if the brain is feeling slow, then your reflexes will be slow, so your ability to save yourself from a car zooming at high speed or to hit the driver who slows down to check you out is, well, dangerously slow. You could land up hurting yourself, and if you are driving a car, then hurting others because of the slow brain to voluntary muscle message. Toh number 1 thing — zinda rahega toh patla hoyega, get it?

So let's summarize what we have learnt till now:

1. Having essential fats as part of your regular diet is crucial for cardio to be an effective fat-burner.
2. Carbs are the primary fuel source for cardio activity, and inadequate carbs in your muscles reduces the body's fat-burning abilities.

Based on this, let's have a detailed look at how to plan your meals, before, during and after cardio.

Technical note — Cardio and dehydration

Wait! Even before we get into meal planning, drink water and loads of it, because cardio is amongst the most dehydrating activities, especially if you train outdoors. Strength training and yoga won't leave you half as dehydrated as cardio will. And sadly only drinking water doesn't help, the more regular you get with cardio, the more actively you have to do 'preventive maintenance' of your hydration status. To put it simply, you have to watch out for dehydrating conditions in your life — stress, air-conditioned offices and processed food is on the list. Stress and overexposure to air-conditioning, you understand (or at least I am going to pretend you do), so will quickly list out some of the processed foods that dehydrate — biscuits (even the ragi and multigrain ones) and other packet food (especially baked variety), alcohol, packaged cereals, colas, energy drinks (even the diet options), buffets and late night meals. These foods and food situations essentially cost your body a lot of water at the cellular level. Now once you start doing preventive maintenance you will have to avoid these foods or food situations at least 48 hours before and after exercise.

Effects of dehydration:	Signs of heat injury because of dehydration:
• Loss of strength from muscles • Decreased workout performance • Reduced cardiac output	• Feeling a chill and standing of hair on ends (piloerection) • Nausea and vomiting • Throbbing headache

Effects of dehydration:	Signs of heat injury because of dehydration:
• Reduced oxygen consumption • Poor thermoregulation • Decreased renal blood flow • Loss of electrolytes • Fast depletion of glycogen	• Dry skin • Unsteadiness and confusion • Anger

I am a doctor and I would like to…

Quite often when I am speaking at an event or a conference and I make 'sweeping statements' like 'you can never get enough water so keep sipping water through the day', etc., invariably there will be some doctor in the crowd who stands up to 'correct' me. All fitness professionals have faced this in their life, the intimidation by doctors, when fear wins over facts. We could be starting out or the best professional in our field or whatever, but doctors get intimidated not by us but I guess by the idea that crowds will listen to something that is not based on fear or staying, as they put it, 'on the safer side'.

'The British Medical Association recommends 8 glasses and anything more than that is harmful to the kidneys', or some such statement will follow. Now number one thing that we should all know is that 8 glasses, whether the British Medical Association said it or anyone else, is at best a generalized statement. Also, to give these associations due credit, they inform people who go by the book that 'hydration requirements change over periods of time and may vary amongst various people / changing environment / medical status / history, etc.' So really, if you must go by these recommendations, then know that what they are telling you is the lowest requirement and not the optimum; they admit to not knowing your life fully and are relying on you to use common sense and drink water accordingly.

Before exercise

4 hours or more prior — The night before or for lunch in case of evening cardio session

Rice-dal-sabzi or sambar-rice-sabzi or roti-sabzi-dal or pulao-raita or your own local version of cereal-pulse-and essential fat like coconut, ghee, filtered ground nut / mustard / sesame oil, that's used for seasoning.

A wholesome meal the night before your training, specially when you train for high-endurance activities like long-distance running, cycling or are a beginner to exercise or if your prime motivation for cardio lies in fat burning, is crucial. A meal that represents local grains, dals, pulses and vegetables along with traditionally used fats (as mentioned above) increases your chances of using fat as a fuel during exercise. This happens because of increased free fatty acids in the blood stream and serves two main purposes: it leads to a slow steady rise in blood sugar so you sleep well through the night (you know how lack of sleep converts to snooze and how that converts to absenteeism from workouts) and allows you to top off liver and glycogen stores.

Pre-workout

Pre-workout meals supply steady blood sugar and delay fatigue. A pre-workout meal must have what you have learnt to recognize as carbs — fruit if exercising in less than 30 minutes, and either poha, upma, idli or paratha, etc., if starting in more than two hours.

During exercise

And what to eat during exercise? Nothing my dear, even if the shelves of your gym are packed with 'cardio blast' or some such product which is a mixture of caffeine, Vitamin B and carbs. Just plain and simple water does the trick of increasing performance and hence calorie burning too. Make sure that you sip and not gulp water. So if you are on a treadmill walking at 6 or running at 8, then slow down to 4 or 6 respectively to sip some water. The reason is that when your breathing and heart rate is higher, it can get tougher for water to make its way to the stomach and then there is always the danger of water entering the windpipe accidently. Even a momentary slow-down makes it easier for the water to make its passage to the stomach. It's exactly this physiological reason why most elderly people will ask you to sit and drink water rather than stand. So slow down and drink, sorry sip, and don't gulp.

And if you run or cycle outdoors and for a long distance, then know that more water and more carb gels or energy drinks is not magically going to make you faster. Energy drinks can get very dense in glucose, and since limited glucose is emptied from the stomach in a short period of time, this (a high concentration of glucose) will retard gastric emptying, leading to less absorption of glucose in the blood, and therefore quicker fatigue. So go slow on energy drinks and stay well hydrated but practise drinking water at every training session, not just on the long runs or race day.

Plain simple glucose or even sugar is enough to give you the 'energy', and so is good old nimbu pani with sugar and kalanamak. (Remember how you keep talking about running being an 'accessible', 'cheap' sport, while wearing shoes that you bought on a 40% discount and cost only 15k?) The deal is to dilute the drink. Technically, it's called **a hypotonic solution, where you can barely taste the 'flavour'**. About 2g or less of glucose per 100ml is a good place to start. OR make nimbu pani and dilute it to 3 times, get it? Now only if dadi ma sold nimbu pani as a 'carb rinser', i.e. something that maintains a balance between gastric emptying and glucose utilization by the working muscle tissue, we would have treated her differently na?

Hyponatremia

The running boom has created this new athlete, the participator and not the competitor. This is the person who runs in double or more of the elite time and has the money and internet access to 'research' every product out there — the belt around the waist carries carb gels, energy drinks, water and then she / he drinks some more water at every 'station'. These are exactly the type of people who are prone to hyponatremia, where sodium levels drop because of excess sweating on one hand and excesses of water and the other 'gels', 'powders', etc. on the other. Symptoms include nausea, headache, vomiting, bloating, and in serious cases, respiratory seizure and coma and can even be fatal. Thankfully in most cases it only means slower performance than 'predicted' and some serious discomfort.

Post exercise

Now post workout, you still need to follow the guidelines that you do post strength training, the 4 R's. And yes, you may not associate protein with cardio but (hold your breath), endurance activity requires much more protein than strength training. Remember the aerobic pathway, remember how all fuels — carb, fat, protein — get converted to Acetyl-CoA? So while running, walking, cycling, swimming, your amino acids also get burned to produce energy (ATP), and unless you replenish those, it is only going to mean loss of the metabolically active tissue of the body, the muscle, which will give you that over-trained, 'I don't want to look like a runner' look. So rehydrate, replenish, repair and recover, and in that order. Don't skip the water and banana and jump straight to protein. In the absence of glycogen, the body converts or breaks down protein to replenish glycogen instead of sparing it for protein purposes, which is repair, maintenance and growth. So don't spend your expensive protein shake on a job that the humble banana can carry out with ease and efficiency. It's not rocket science, it's chemistry (another of my fav lines, this time from *Breaking Bad*).

Anyway, let's just recap:

Pre workout	**How it helps**
1. The night before or 4-6 hours earlier Dal-rice-sabzi with ghee / roti-sabzi-dal with ghee / Poha / Upma / Paratha / Idli-chutney-sambar Wholesome, regional, traditional meal with carbs, protein and essential fats	• Slow steady rise in blood sugar • Allows the body to optimize liver and muscle glycogen stores • Essential fats teach the body to preferentially burn the FFA (free fatty acids) during exercise • Puts your mind in 'workout mode' versus snooze mode • Delays fatigue during exercise
2. About 30 mins before exercise Fresh fruit – anything seasonal Banana preferable for intense exercises or exercise in warm conditions	• Allows you to top off liver glycogen stores • Ensures that blood sugars are at optimum • Allows the body a smooth transition to fat burning within minutes of exercise
During exercise 1. Indoors and not more than 50 mins of workout • Plain room temperature or cool water • Sip intermittently. Slow down and sip, don't gulp	• Allows the working muscle to contract without cramping • Better thermoregulation • Prevents heat injury
2. Longer than 60 mins and outdoors Hypotonic or diluted nimbu pani or glucose water with salt (use unprocessed salt for better ratio of Na and K – the two main electrolytes of the body)	• Has a protective effect on the vital organs – heart and kidneys • Delays fatigue and ensures optimum fat burning

<table>
<tr><td>Post workout
Follow the 4 R.
Rehydrate. Replenish.
Repair. Recover
Water. Carb. Protein.
Antioxidants
* For long runs – potato sandwich is a great idea. Carry it with you and have the protein shake after getting home.</td><td>• Allows the body to shift from catabolism to anabolism
• Brings back the electrolyte balance of the body
• Prevents the body from slipping into a hypoglycaemic state
• Quicker glycogen replenishment
• Prevents muscle tissue breakdown and accelerates recovery
• Antioxidants keep the free radical damage in check
• Lessens tissue damage and other aesthetic issues like tanning, break-outs etc.</td></tr>
</table>

Inability to fuel the body correctly invariably comes in the way of exercise performance. Not just in how many calories you will burn but also in terms of whether you will be able to take exercise to the next level, and whether you will keep up with your planned frequency or just make a donation to the gym / exercise class / shoe store without even gaining the 80cc benefit.

Chapter Summary

Cardio facts

- Exercise lowers the resting heart rate and improves heart health
- Both aerobic and anaerobic exercises are needed to improve heart health
- Heart and lung, the involuntary organs, are much stronger than the TBLJ and muscles
- So to train / improve heart health, it's imperative that the muscles need to be trained / used
- So to make progress in your cardio exercise, you will need to weight train. This will have the following benefits:
    - Strengthen TBLJ and the muscles and allow them to bear more forces
    - Allow you to stimulate the anaerobic pathway, which influences and improves your cardio-respiratory fitness and therefore VO_2 max and lactate threshold
    - Train your body to preferentially use fat as a source aerobically and spare glycogen for the anaerobic pathway.
- Training at LT / AT will help increase both speed and stamina by pushing the lactate threshold farther
- You can use the FITT formula and the training diary as tools to make / record progress in cardio
- Along with carbs and proteins, it is imperative to add essential fats to your diet so that cardio becomes a fat-burning activity

- Staying hydrated and preventive maintenance of your hydration status is crucial for cardio
- Use hypotonic solutions during long duration cardio activity

Cardio Fads

1. Mixing cardio or aerobic with dance or martial arts, typically done as group classes

That's nice as a break but not as the backbone of the entire training program or even just 'cardio'. Group activity is definitely fun so do it by all means, but also train aerobically with running / cycling / swimming or anything else of your choice. The limitation with group classes is that they don't necessarily operate or function at your individual fitness levels. So you may end up either overtraining or under-training crucial fitness parameters of strength, flexibility and endurance. Then there is also the 'shame factor': 'shit! The fat aunty can do it and I can't', or versions of this, so safety gets overlooked.

Now you really want to dance? Dance na? Wanna kick? By all means go for it! Want to learn how the Zen masters held their thighs while standing, please, go ahead. Want to learn the south Indian martial art kalaripayattu? Why not, do it. But what is this obsession with 'mixing' it up and upping the calorie burn, etc. Martial art and dance forms are worthy of practising out of purity and passion and not with the greediness of losing weight. This whole 'mixing' leads to loss of traditional sequencing or choreography of these forms of dance and martial art and leads only to sweat and not glory. Come on, there is so much more out there beyond the calorie burn.

Zumba

By the way, Zumba was born out of the fact that the main instructor forgot his tapes, so he made do with whatever he had and 'mixed' various dance, martial arts and squat / lunge kind of movements to the beat of music. Because he was a good choreographer, the class loved it. Over a period of time, this was further improvised, and various other elements and stuff like 'toning, strengthening' were added, but essentially it was born as a nice break from the regular workout and let us just keep it like that. Also, if you really are a fan then on your trip abroad forget the usual 'so much you walk' and take a Zumba class, ensure that the instructor is of African origin and trust me you will realize what paani kum chai your Zumba back home is ;).

2. Cardio on an empty stomach 'to burn fat'

We have already discussed the importance of carbs in your meal prior to a workout session. So just convert this to 'cardio after early dinner and on a light stomach.' See, let me just say it, if you are really fat, it took mehnat to get there, right? I mean, you didn't get there overnight, it's years of eating a certain way (not eating anything for the longest time and once you start eating not knowing where to stop), not working out, not really being very active (you have solid reasons for that I am sure), but the fact is here you are, after years of neglecting yourself. And when self-neglect sets in, the body forgets how to burn fat or at least how to preferentially burn fat over the other readily-available fuels. And if it took years to collect fat, it is going to take you months to lose it. Cardio on an empty stomach may lead to fat-burning in a super trained athlete whose body knows how to burn fat, but in your and my body it only means low-calorie output, more fatigue and sacrifice of that precious fat-burning muscle tissue. So no, no cardio on an empty stomach, at least not till you have been consistent with training for 3 years, ok?

3. Cardio before lifting weights

Now this should be really simple — no cardio ever before strength training. See cardio can use glycogen (carbs), fat and protein as fuel to produce muscular contractions and allow you to move forward. But weight training can only use glycogen as it lies in the anaerobic zone (and I am assuming here that your reps are now 8-12 and not 'high'). Now if you have already exhausted or even reduced your glycogen stores with that 10 or 20 minutes of whatever you do on the treadmill before going into the weights section, it's like wanting your body to run on a low or zero tank.

Obviously you will end up lifting less or nothing close to your body's ability to exert muscular force. In effect you will burn less calories during the strength / weight training session (due to less fuel there will be less muscle fibre recruitment) and that will have an effect on the after-burn. Very simply, the less the intensity of your workout in the anaerobic zone, the less the fat-burning benefit or after-burn post exercise.

Why does your trainer still ask you to do cardio then? Well mostly because all their clients turn up late and they don't know how to say no to so many people. So even if you turn up for your 11 a.m. session at 11 a.m. you are on the treadmill for 20 minutes coz your trainer is finishing up with the earlier client who came in late. It's a logistical and not a physiological adjustment that you are making here. Also, instead of noon, you finish little later and never bother asking your trainer why your session gets extended daily. You are trained to feel that if you paid for 1 hour and got 1.20 hours, it is somehow better; it is not, at least not for your fat-burning.

On the other hand are trainers who train you for 30 to 40 minutes and then put you on the treadmill for 20 to 30 minutes so that you feel that you worked out for an hour. This again is not required, and you have learnt that weight training should get over in less than 60 minutes in the strength training chapter. But in terms of fuel availability, it is still better than doing cardio before weights (of course it's not ideal).

Cardio FAQs

Q: What is better, running on the road or treadmill?

A: What is better, wearing a pink tee-shirt or a yellow one? Depends on what you prefer, right? Choose between treadmill and road depending on what makes you feel better and makes you feel like you put your time to good use. Personally, I like to run on a treadmill and cycle on the road. That's because, well, I just prefer it like that ;-). Just make sure that your treadmill is of good quality and is regularly serviced.

And if there is a hierarchy regarding what is better for your weight-bearing joints, then here goes: Sand. Grass. Even mud path. And then come the treadmill or road. Some high-funda treadmills now have inbuilt cushioning so they are slightly better than roads.

Q: *I always get a headache / sinus attack post cardio or aerobic workout or long run / walks.*

A: Wow! That makes you a walking -talking hypoglycaemic and heat-injured athlete. Sip on water during exercise and post exercise whether it was indoors or outdoors, have a diluted salt-glucose drink or the diluted nimbu pani and follow it up with the 4 R's. Also do a longer warm-up and a proper cool down before and after exercise. Till the condition settles, lower both the intensity and duration of your workout and work on building it up slowly over a few weeks.

Q: *After long runs I am miles away from any post-workout meal. Any suggestions?*

A: Carry dry dates and some raisins in your pocket and have that the minute you cool down and during stretching. My personal favourite option for long runs is a potato sandwich. Keep it in your car or at the place where you do your stretching; eat it as soon as you are done stretching and definitely before heading back home, the last thing you want is an accident / injury post the long run, and it's a meal that fits into the 4 R's perfectly well. Get home, and before you shower, read the newspaper, etc., have your protein shake.

Q: *How about running without shoes?*

A: If you are not a trained athlete, which means that if you run a marathon in 4 hours or more and a half marathon in 2 hours or more then, no, don't even think about it. Shoes are crucial for the cushioning your feet and your weight-bearing joints require to carry your body weight for all the time it takes to finish your run. Walk around at home barefoot instead, and you can also be barefoot on sand, grass, but on roads — shoes please.

Q: *Realistically I can spare only two days to work out, what do you suggest?*

A: Well, definitely do your strength training, and to ensure that you don't completely ignore cardio, you can do an easy run or cycle for 20 minutes post strength training on the upper body day. Because during weights you will utilize your glycogen, even if the stores are going down or exhausted post exercise, it is not a limiting fuel for cardio as it can use or burn fat too and can keep you going post weights. That way you are progressively overloading the aerobic energy or pathway too without making the investment of another day.

Q: *I find cardio very boring so I avoid it and only do weight training but then sometimes I think, what about my heart health?*

A: Well, if you are seriously into weight training and lift respectable weights on your compound exercises for the large muscle groups — legs, back and chest — then know that those raise your heart rate and breathing too. Weight training may not be popular for its 'heart benefits', but it surely offers them to you. So don't worry, your heart is not complaining or shrinking in size because of the choice of exercise. Also know that cardio turns 'boring' because of the lack of challenge or overload on the aerobic pathway. If you learn to use the FITT principle and the exercise log, I am sure that even cardio will turn into an activity that you look forward to.

Q: *I am following the Kenyan athletes training program for the marathon this year, is that ok?*

A: The Kenyan training program or following any elite runner's program is a mistake because you have completely overlooked your current fitness levels. Most Kenyan runners have a history of running from school to home, village to village and sometimes even running to save their lives, you have almost never been in any of those situations. When they do hill runs for strength, or train 3 times a day for endurance, know that they have the body weight, the strength, speed, agility, VO_2 max, etc., to cope with or adapt to this stimuli. For us city slickers, running every day can also be harmful. So stick to the basics, rotate or alternate the energy systems you choose to overload on any particular day, get a day of strength training, spare a day for stretching and resting and don't run more than 10% of what you ran the previous week. And yes, run for the joy of it, and run without risking injuries.

Q: *How do I keep up while travelling?*

A: Boss pehla toh are you 'keeping up' while not travelling? Because if you are, then just chill when you are travelling, walk around the place you're in, it's a good way to get to know it, its people and culture, and a good break from the routine of 'burning calories'. And if you travel on business and have no time to walk around, then how about making time for a nice massage, because relaxing and doing nothing is also essentially fat-burning in nature. Aerobic pathway, remember?

The problem with strength training is, most hotel gyms are poorly equipped and rarely serviced, often receiving step-motherly treatment of being either in the basement or in a dingy corner. The least paid guy in the hotel industry is probably the gym trainer, so forget about getting someone to 'spot' you. I have this problem with 'clubs' too, I mean they are supposed to spread the 'fitness culture', but it's the banquets that face the gardens and swimming pools and the gyms are invariably in the basement and with treadmills facing walls or mirrors.

All right, if you really must do something, how about practising yoga asanas, and if nothing else, a nice round of suryanamaskar? Learn to do them right first, under a good teacher, while you are not travelling. And with that, let's move on to the yoga chapter ☺.

Chapter 5

Yoga — Rethink and Relearn

To be consumers of yoga, or students of yoga, the choice is yours.
– BKS Iyengar

A short history of yoga

Once upon a time, India was a land of sages and rishis who practised yoga as a way of life. No one went to classes then, and yoga didn't have fancy names or a multimillion-dollar industry attached to it or promises of quickly fixing your stress, backache, asthma or whatever else. Everyone practised yoga in their own way and asana practice formed a small but integral part of their dinacharya, or daily routine.

Much later, but still a long time ago, when Mahmud of Ghazni raided India, he was advised by his trusted aide Al-Beruni to not touch the scriptures on yoga, or to not touch them at least till they were translated into Arabic. This, thought Al-Beruni, who came down to India as part of the Ghazni gang, was as precious or more crucial than looting jewels and adding India to the empire. Proficient in many languages and with a deep understanding of Islam and its true values, Al-Beruni's job in India was to learn Sanskrit and understand its culture for two reasons: (a) India's deep-rooted and holistic culture was both respected and seen as a threat to the invasion (not its military powers or lack of them), and (b) anything in this rich culture that was worthy of adopting was to be translated and taken back home.

The first translation of Patanjali's *Yoga Sutras,* then, was into Arabic, and that is how yoga got its first foreign following; this was long before the 'My dear brothers and sisters' speech by Swami Vivekananda. Till date Al-Beruni's translation is regarded as the best and the most authentic one — the Persian and Islamic culture had the richness and depth to accommodate the 196 Sanskrit verses, and the translator had the deep understanding and practice of pursuing anything including asana, pranayama, etc., religiously.

So, even as the Mughals translated and took the wisdom of yoga with them, back home it started vanishing from daily life — pushed away into the high Himalaya or remote villages. By the time Swami Vivekananda made the epic speech at Chicago that attracted Western following to yogic wisdom, the British had already implemented a 'modern' education system. This system had no room for asana practice in daily life, there was no effort to control or discipline the senses, purity of thought, breath, body were not measures of progress, and success was not to be found in the knowledge of purusha and prakriti.

Education acquired a new meaning and degrees were your ladder to success (money, recognition, etc.). Everything indigenous, including yoga as a way of life, was systematically rooted out and a new system, new values, new language were introduced to 'reform' us. We were all to become 'Macaulay's children', conditioned to look up to the West and follow their ideals and in turn look down upon ours. The process of weeding out the Indian way of life and Indian education system, with its focus on maths, astronomy, Sanskrit, yoga, philosophy, and a holistic way of life (that was already in place up to university level), had started way back in 1835, the speech came only in 1893. Al-Beruni was actually quite upset with his Badshaah for so ruthlessly demolishing temples, sculptures and the culture that thrived on yogic vidya. He didn't get a chance to see how ruthless the British invaders were and how one could manipulate an entire culture and belief system without causing any 'in your face' destruction.

Anyway, history is not my subject and I write only from the point of view of a sports nutritionist / fitness consultant who lives and watches the continued daily destruction of this all-encompassing vidya into a quick fix 'get rid of your bulge', 'see white light', 'improve flexibility', 'learn pranayama from TV', 'get enlightened in 3 weeks of classes' and the like. Honestly, **our impatience and ignorance along with our ability to buy into quick-fixes and our willingness to be fooled is a force that defeats the might and malice of both the British and the Mughul invaders.** Ghazni and Macaulay pale in comparison to the way we destroy our heritage and traditional wisdom.

So what am I saying? Yoga is not going to give you weight loss? See! You always knew that! Saala, fukat mein book pe paisa waste kiya! No, I am saying that it will give you way more than weight loss or a glowing complexion. It will give you insight, innocence and intelligence to see the world and yourself as constantly changing and impermanent beings. It will become the guiding force you live by, a force that tells you that the body ages, you don't, so that Botox is really unnecessary ☺.

But yoga survives

As 'education' further wiped out this practice or whatever of it remained in our daily lives, it survived nevertheless, in our homes and in our hearts; in a vehry vehry filmi way — once you have internalized a practice, once it has been imprinted on your heart / DNA, it mysteriously and uncannily finds a way to carry itself forward and to express itself in the most unusual places. Look at your grandparents' wedding photos or portraits (hopefully you have some): the man always stands to the right of the lady. The reason is that male energy or prana flows through the right nostril and the feminine energy or apana flows through the left. Even the way they pose for pictures is rooted in yogic wisdom; so is the way they eat, the way they want to live and most importantly the way they want to die (amongst family and grandchildren — after fulfilling every duty, without being a financial / emotional burden on the family). All of it can be traced to the imprint this vidya left on our hearts. In pure yogic terms, it's called the 'sanskara', the deep grooves it forms in our minds that get transmitted from generation to generation.

This imprint is just one of the many boons of a life that abides by the law of ahimsa, non-injury. It's such a central theme of the Indian way of life that it forms the prime-most 'Yama', the laws of self-restraint that one must follow to lead a yogic life.

The schools of yoga

Today of course we confuse yoga with some form of physical exercise or some quick weight loss aid or something that celebrities do. In fact I think we can roughly divide India in two parts: one that thinks Patanjali is someone they see on TV and the other that buys designer tracks to go to yoga classes taught by Caucasian women with exotic names. But there's a third India, which tucks the tee-shirt inside and practises in ventilated rooms with hard floors, with teachers who look and behave like regular people, no halo around their heads, no exotic names, no orange robes, just hardcore disciplinarians who believe in living their art. This variety usually belongs to one of the classical schools of yoga who try and keep up with the essence of *Hatha Yoga Pradipika* and Patanjali's *Yoga Sutras*, the two guiding texts of yogic philosophy and practice.

As yoga started moving deep into the Himalaya, the masters taught the vidya to their students and instructed them to pass it on only to 'deserving' students. Deserving students essentially meant students who practised with dispassion, without the temptation of 'result', with devotion, who spent time contemplating the meaning of the practice and showed the genius of putting their art to practice. Needless to say, deserving students were hard to come by and slowly but surely some of the techniques, practices, rituals, etc. died with the teacher; this was considered higher (better) than letting the great vidya, so meticulously practised and treasured, fall in the wrong hands and get diluted or distorted. You can partly see this with tantra yoga being mistaken as casual sex when its true meaning lies in something very different and beyond physical sex.

Patanjali and Ashtanga yoga

Patanjali, the saint who lived long before any invasion took place, documented and codified the yogic wisdom from various practices prevalent at those times into eight clear steps (in his *Yoga Sutras*), and called it the 'Ashta-anga' yoga, the eight branches / folds or bodies of yoga. This remains till date a very clear and practical step-by-step guideline to help you progress in your yoga practice.

The Ashtanga or the 8 limbs of yoga as described by sage Patanjali:

1. Yama (Self-restraints). There are 5 yamas:
   - Ahimsa – Non-violence
   - Satya – Truthfulness
   - Asteya – Non stealing
   - Bramhacharya – Divine conduct
   - Apargraha – Non hoarding
2. Niyam (Observances). There are 5 niyams:
   - Saucha – Cleanliness
   - Santosha – Contentment
   - Tapas – Disciplined approach
   - Swadhyaya – Self study
   - Ishavaraparidhan – Surrender to God
3. Asana – Disciplining the body using postures
4. Pranayama – Expansion and discipline of the breath
5. Pratyahara – Withdrawal of senses
6. Dharana – Concentration
7. Dhyana – Meditation
8. Samadhi – One with the true self

So let's just speak of what happened to asanas — of the 84 lakh asanas (an asana each from every kind), less than 84 survive today, and most of us can't even do and don't know the names of a dozen of these surviving asanas. The two gurus who managed to carry the torch and pass it on to their students world over and influence what we understand of yoga today are Swami Sivananda of Rishikesh and Krishnamacharya of Mysore. Almost all teachers who teach with the whole 'no frills attached' attitude can in fact be traced to one of these two lineages. However, to say that these two were the only ones would be incorrect and limited. There are many gurus who taught the essence and it survives and thrives through their schools, be it the Ramkrishna mission, Chinmayananda, Swami Rama's ashram, and many other institutes.

Here is a brief overview of the main students of Swami Sivananda and Krishnamacharya and the schools of yoga they established:

Teacher / Lineage	Students – Schools of yoga
Swami Sivananda	Swami Satyananda – Bihar School of Yoga
	Swami Vishnudevananda – Yoga Vedanta Forest Academy
	Swami Chidananda – Divine Life Society, Rishikesh
Krishnamacharya	Pattabhi Jois – Ashtanga or Mysore style
	BKS Iyengar – Yoga with props, main centre in Pune
	Desikarchar – Vini yoga or Nada yoga, centre in Chennai

The two main gurus are called many things, like Krishnamacharya is called 'the father of modern yoga', but irrespective of names, they represent the collective yoga wisdom that existed in India. And their teaching continues to influence what's happening in the yoga studio next door, whether you are in Santa Cruz or San Jose!

To further your understanding of the schools of yoga and to make it easier for you to choose, I have summarized their working, their specialties if you want to call it that. Note that this comes from my very limited understanding and biases, known and unknown.

Yoga School	Main Centre	Specialty / Known for
Yoga Vedanta Forest Academy – Swami Vishnudevananda	Neyyar Dam, Kerala	• 12 basic postures that are easy to follow • Pranayama taught in every class • Chanting encouraged • Teacher training course – 1 month • Advance course – 1 month • Continuous training available across centres
Bihar School of Yoga – Swami Satyananda	Munger, Bihar	• Best known for its yoga literature • Every book is worth buying • Initiated women into sanyasa • Taught and propagated use of yoga nidra (even taught to jail inmates as part of reform) • Basic course – 4 months • Continuous training available in Munger, Bihar

Yoga School	Main Centre	Specialty / Known for
Divine Life Society – Swami Chidananda	Rishikesh, Uttarakhand	• Strong base of Vedanta and philosophy • Teaches and promotes sadhana as a way of life • Conducts talks daily – open to all • Anyone can go and meditate, chant in the halls • Runs medical facilities, orphanage, educational institutes • Has 1- and 2-month courses but only for men
Ashtanga – Pattabhi Jois	Mysore, Karnataka	• Style known as Mysore / Ashtanga / Vinayasa yoga • Dynamic flow from one asana into another with the breath • Probably the most popular form of yoga • Suryanamaskars are taught as the foundation of the practice • Practice broken down to 6 series and students progress at their own pace • New asanas introduced only after students perfect each posture in a given series • No certification courses offered, students have to go to Mysore and learn • Dedicated students and serious practitioners can lead class as a teacher

Yoga School	Main Centre	Specialty / Known for
Iyengar yoga – BKS Iyengar	Pune, Maharashtra	• Known for precision in asanas • Makes use of 'props' – belts, ropes, bricks, benches, chairs to make asanas accessible to all • Challenging classes and strict teachers • Doesn't teach pranayama until student is considered ready by teacher • Offers certification abroad but in India, students handpicked to teach • Indian teachers will have 8 or more years of practise • Abroad, about 2-3 years to get certification • All teachers visit Pune to learn from senior teachers under the eagle eye of BKS Iyengar • Solid modules of therapeutic yoga
Nada yoga – Desikarchar	Chennai, Tamil Nadu	• Style also known as Vini yoga • Combines asana with chanting • Special courses offered on Vedic chanting • Offers courses of varying time, including a 2- or 3-year diploma

Choosing the right yoga school for you — a checklist

This book is not meant to be a step-by-step guide of how to get into a yoga posture, there are some superb ones out there and if you really want to lay your hands on the best one, it's

Light on Yoga, or the easier version, *Illustrated Light on Yoga* by BKS Iyengar. I am here to tell you how to look out for yourself, to help you choose a yoga school that most appeals to your temperament and liking, to allow you to make an informed choice so that you may continue your practice without being injured or misled. So I am going to try and list down a few things that an honest yoga school will always do or won't do. Think of this as a checklist of considerations before joining a yoga class:

Will	Will not
Ask you to give details of health and medical history	Promise quick cures at the end of a certain number of sessions
Ask you to wear comfortable clothing	Make it compulsory to wear certain colours or brands for 'optimum benefits'
Ask you to eat a light meal before class – either a fruit or 2-3 hour gap after a meal	Ask you to come on an empty stomach or have unrealistic meal gaps (4 hours and above)
Encourage you to eat home-cooked, local, seasonal including all grains	Encourage soups, salads or any diet plans based on avoiding carbs and counting calories
Make it clear that asanas are essential part of wellbeing and evolution	Look down upon asanas
Believe that pranayama done wrongly can harm more than bring any good	Promote pranayama for quick enlightenment

Will	Will not
Believe that you need to first prepare your body and breath for meditation	Teach that meditation will show you lights (camera and action)
Teacher practises what she/he preaches	Have teachers that behave like gyaanis / realized souls
Class is ventilated and clean	Have classes that are either too cold or too hot
You will be encouraged to walk straight	Encourage you to walk with a halo
Kapalbhati will be taught as a kriya and with a lot of discretion	Reduce kapalbhati to a must-do exercise for losing the paunch
Class sequence based on the effect asanas have on the subtle body	Have a class sequence based on various body parts — chest, back, arms, abs, thighs, etc.

Typically, yoga schools that are high on integrity will also have a few basics in place. They:

- Will emphasize on following the yama and niyama
- Promote asanas as an essential step to the vast science of yoga
- Teach that asanas can be taken up at any age, any stage, any gender and at any phase of the menstrual cycle
- Teach pranayama as a serious practice and after proficiency in asana is gained; you will be made to understand that it requires attention to detail or it may harm

- Teach that it's easy to access pranayama and pratyahara through asanas
- Teach that dhyana, dharana and samadhi cannot be forced or achieved by mere sitting and 'focusing', these require grace and practise of the basics — yama, niyama and asana
- Will not ask you for money / donation / favours over and above what is being charged as class fee
- Even though may take therapy or special classes for certain conditions ranging from back ache to cancer, will never sell a certain asana for a certain condition and will make it amply clear that all asanas are necessary for all conditions, including the condition of wellbeing
- Will encourage you to practise and work hard in every class
- Will not promote any fads including fasting
- Will not use terms like 'kapha, vata, pitta' frivolously
- Will have teachers who know enough to know that they don't know enough

---

Technical note — Yoga and energy systems

Now it is tough, almost impossible, to classify yoga as purely or even dominantly as either aerobic or anaerobic. In fact most Eastern or classical disciplines, be it dance, music, martial art or yoga asanas are both aerobic and anaerobic even within the same movement. Like a young dancer may take up to a year to learn all the adavus (basic steps) of Bharatnatyam, but with required practise and proficiency, she can effortlessly perform all adavus in one single hour. Then she will also learn to do the same adavus in at least three different speeds — slow, medium and fast — and by doing that learn to create the same movement using different types of muscle fibres, fuel substrates and energy systems.

Asanas are similar: the posture in which you struggle and your quads shiver will turn into your go-to asana to release your back after a long drive or a flight. The sirsasana which was impossible and 'freaky' just a few years ago turns into your resting posture or your 'come home, lounge on the sofa, switch channels' routine turns to 'get into sirsasana, then to sarvangasana and finish with paschimotanasana' routine. The sirsasana against a wall and in the centre of the room will utilise different energy systems as the muscles undergo different loading. Asana practice, like the classical system of dance, goes through various rhythms and even posture sequence, based on things like season. So yoga can't really be qualified as any particular energy system.

The only 'energy' that yoga talks about is the prana shakti, the divine life force, and harmonizing its flow in the body to bring about the wellbeing of mankind and his surroundings. Yoga asanas utilize and activate all the energetic pathways and muscle fibre types, the purpose is to turn the body into an instrument that is in a condition to achieve the highest purpose of life, Samadhi. Because of the intelligent planning of asanas, their sequence and their ability to lend themselves to different seasons and fitness levels and genders and across age groups, asana practice is often thought of as a physical exercise that brings about improvement of flexibility, strength and stamina levels, but while that is true, the purpose remains quite different.

Yoga in practice

The sequence of asanas

The asana practice in the traditional schools of yoga will have some basic rules:

- Come to class only after a bath
- Wear comfy clothing that doesn't make you awkward in any posture including inversions
- Follow an ageless sequence the basis of which is pranic flow through the chakras (subtle energy centres of the body). Here is a generic one:

Sequence	Asanas	Effects
Prayer	To Patanjali *Hatha Yoga Pradipika* Saraswati or Ganesha Sahanavavatu Om Invoking name of God	• Bringing the focus to the practice of asana • Dedicating practice to a higher reality • Asking for grace before practice
Warm-up	Suptapadangusthasana Suryanamaskar Uttanasana Adhomukhasvanasana Variety of standing postures like – trikonasana / virabhadrasana	• Awaken the mind and senses • Increase blood flow to the periphery • Prepare for the practice
Inversions	These will usually follow the basic sequence – *Sirsasana Sarvangasana Halasana *Beginner classes may teach sirsasana at the very end or not teach it initially	• Learning to stand on your head / shoulders • Involving underused neuro-muscular pathways • Overcoming conditioning / convention

Sequence	Asanas	Effects
Forward bends	Paschimotanasana Janu sirasasana Prasarita padottanasana Marichayasana 1	• Improving flexibility of the lower back and hamstrings • Learning to let go • Creating awareness of the back body (often ignored)
Back bends	Dhanurasana Bhujangasana Ustrasana Setubandhasana	• Improving strength in the spine and back muscles • Breaking through insecurity and fear • Improving health of digestive organs
Twists	Ardha matsyendrasana Bharadwajasana Parsvakonasana Anantasana	• Increasing and maintaining mobility of the spine • Churning out the physical and mental toxins • Improving blood sugar control and fertility
Balancing asana	Kakasana Mayurasana Vrksasana Ardhachandrasana	• Improves strength of the core muscle groups • Learning to uplift while being grounded • Creating a sense of balance in the mind and body

Sequence	Asanas	Effects
Restorative asana	Supta virasana Supta badha konasana Viparit karani Savasana	• Relaxes the body and the mind • Anti-ageing and stress-busters in nature • Restores the blood circulation, breath and lowers the heart rate

Ok, now this was tough for me to write given the fact that this remains a very gross and physical way of breaking down postures that encompass a philosophy that has influenced, enriched and given direction to an entire culture, belief and value system. But then, it's a well-established fact that everything that is profound must be a simple and practical approach. **Asanas form those simple steps to gaining more profound direction in life.**

The thing you must remember is the list above is indicative and not exhaustive. You must also know that asana is a method of gaining access to the otherwise inaccessible and impenetrable aspects of our existence — the subtle and the causal bodies. Another very crucial aspect that you must understand is that the structure above can be taught based on the level of the class (and teacher), your medical history, season, region, gender, age, insight: entirely standing, sitting, lying down, on a chair / bench, hospital bed, with belts, bolsters, trees, grass, supine, prone, etc. Not trying to confuse you but just informing you that asanas are across the globe for a reason — they aren't limited by a set number and style of postures and can be endlessly adapted and taught across all fitness levels.

Other factors that influence the sequence of asanas:

Season: My teacher would get us to spend less time in sirsasana and more time in sarvangasana when it got hotter in Mumbai, like in May. We did more forward bends and just about did a mild backward bend, as forward bends can cool off the body and ease the effects of the summer heat on us.

Menstruation: No inversions as it disrupts the natural flow of the uterine mucus and more focus on forward bends and restorative asanas.

Feeling low and down: He would get me to do setubandhasana on a bench or a brick to increase blood flow to my brain so that I would feel more alert / energetic and at the same time help lower my heart rate and make my breathing deeper.

Jet lag or recovery from a tired day: Viparit karani so that my lower body recycled its toxins, the digestive system felt nourished and the heart rate slowed down. Btw, will share a secret: do this just before wearing a short dress so that the knees look sharp, thighs toned and cheeks flushed.

Example: A beginner's sequence

When you begin, the sequence — the warm-up, inversion, forward bend, backward bend, twist, balance — will be taught standing up. You will almost never sit, the teacher will try and have you access your sense of balance, agility, strength while standing up and build the routine from there. For example:

- *Adhomukhasvanasana* will become the inversion instead of sirsasana or sarvangasana.
- *Prasarita padotanasana* will be the forward bend.
- *Uttanasana or adhomukhasvanasana* will be used to access the muscles which are used in backward bends
- *Parshvakonasana* will be the twist and the tree pose or *vrikshasana* the balance.
- Your teacher may finally have you lying down in the *savasana* or may use the *uttanasana* as the restorative pose to end the class.
- The same sequence can be done sitting, lying down prone or supine; essentially the same postures lend themselves to training you to access different muscle groups and neuromuscular pathways depending on whether you are trying to use it as a forward bend, twist or a restorative asana — for example *janusirsasana.*

Example — Sequence of 12 basic postures as taught in Sivananda style

1. Sirsasana (headstand)
2. Sarvangasana (shoulder stand)
3. Halasana (plough)
4. Matsyasana (fish)
5. Paschimotanasana (sitting forward bend)
6. Bhujangasana (cobra)
7. Salabhasana (locust pose)
8. Dhanurasana (bow pose)
9. Ardha Matysendrasana (half spinal twist)
10. Kakasana (crow pose)

11. Padahastasana (standing forward bend)
12. Trikonasana (triangle pose)

Savasana (dead man pose)

Meal planning for yoga

Yoga philosophy believes that food makes our physical body, the annamaya kosha, and this goes on to influence our mana, mind. I am sure you have noticed how the mind dances from desire to anger to fatigue after you have eaten a chocolate pastry or dug into a tub of ice cream late in the night. And just one recollection of your late night drama will prove that food does influence both the body and the mind, so I will rest my case and focus on what really matters — the logistics.

Yoga emphasizes on pure food; that which is fresh, local, seasonal and even ethically grown. The belief is that food is God itself, and should ultimately reach the person who sees God within, outside and as an all-pervading, omnipresent entity. So basically yoga is way beyond the number of calories you ate and whether or not you made it to the class on an empty stomach. It's about **realizing that it is food that makes every experience in this physical body possible**. Without food there is no body, no mind, no intellect, no memory, no ability to see, hear, touch, smell things. It is food that makes physical, and therefore spiritual, progress possible, so one must not just eat food but view every experience around food with a sense of responsibility, devotion actually. Eating with devotion is the exact opposite of raiding the fridge because you are bored, or drinking coffee because you are sleepy. So if any amount of suryanamaskars or 'dying in yoga class' is not making you thin, then think about how and why you are eating.

Eating with a sense of devotion ensures that you are more in tune with the body's natural rhythm and understand when to eat and where to stop eating. Basically **eat for nourishment and not entertainment, eat for the intelligence and not indulgence.**

Ya, I know I said food logistics. So here goes:

Before class: Stay light on the stomach.

Yeah light, not empty. Now, without food you are gonna collapse in class and blame it on ardhachandrasana or sirsasana. I don't know from where this whole 'empty stomach' funda came from. None of the traditional schools ask you to practise on an empty stomach, but they do ask you to take dinner around sunset. So if you are eating dinner around 7 p.m., or because you are really working till late, at around 9 p.m., and then waking up by 7ish for a yoga class, it is totally cool (actually recommended) that you have some dry fruit / fruit / some milk (without any additions — only sugar, honey, jaggery is ok) about 20 to 30 minutes before class.

This whole 'empty stomach' business I think is propagated by people doing full throttle 'pranayama' or 'meditation' in the morning. Where basically the minute they sit for their 'practice' they begin to fear that the maid won't turn up, fantasize about the neighbour, brood over a memory that's 25 years old and eventually lose total track of why they are sitting on a mat in the first place. Mostly this empty stomach means it has had a chai or coffee on rising and even if it hadn't had these stimulants, it's still processing the late night dinner.

So these thoughts are coming because of the undigested food material in the GI tract, the bane of an indisciplined lifestyle. If you do fall in this category, take your dinner at least an hour earlier, don't watch TV post dinner, and know that meditation and pranayama require much more than sitting cross-legged. Be ready to work on the basics. And the basics are Yama, self-restraint, the most important one being mitahar, eating in a state of balance, coz without balance there is no yoga.

Pre-class meal options:

Morning class: Fruit / dry fruit / milk, if it's first thing in the morning.

Mid-morning class: An hour or two post a wholesome, home-cooked breakfast.

Afternoon class: Schedule the class 2 to 3 hours post lunch (and no smoking / tea / coffee post lunch).

Evening class: Eat a fruit before leaving from office and on your way to class. It will give you enough stability in the stomach to perform asanas but not slow you down in class.

Late night class: I mean, really? Ok, I don't know what you are into, but 4 hours post dinner as digestion is slower post sunset.

Post class: Have a wholesome meal.

Water: Always start with a glass of water that you sip on while sitting and not while standing or running towards your car. The yogic belief is that water forms our breath. So drinking water is like a pranayama practice, and just like you can't rush through pranayama, you sit for it with certain protocol, you should accord the same treatment to water.

Post-class meal options:

Fresh, seasonal, local and purified by fire (cooked) meals are the best option. So either poha / upma / paratha / homemade porridge of local millets or grains or rice-dal-sabzi / roti-sabzi-dahi are good options depending on the time of the day.

When — You can eat almost immediately post yoga class and unless there is a HUGE travel time between class and home, go home and eat. Avoid carrying meals to class.

The squatty potty

In 1999 when I finished my PG in Sports Science and Nutrition, Appa (my grandfather) couldn't fathom what I was actually going to do for a living. When I tried telling him, everything that came out of my mouth sounded really stupid – basically versions of 'tell people what to eat, help them get more active'. 'Shit outside and eat at home, that's all they need to do! Why should anyone even have to ask you?' Appa wondered!

'Parsakade', I am going towards the back (going to the fields), is how his family and basically everyone from Konkan would describe 'potty time'. They would walk out towards the field, a nice walk in the open by the trees and overlooking the hills and relieve themselves every morning. They had no dirty word for it like shishi, poopoo, potty, sandas, nothing, just a walk to the back. Now physiologically, this little walk to the back would stimulate the gastrocolic response or reflex, where there is a natural urge to eliminate waste from the large intestines and make room in the stomach to receive more food. Wow! Isn't that a great way to start your day, physiologically primed to make the most of your morning meal? A clear stomach is a priceless joy and keeps the potential of either lifting you out of misery or making you feel miserable. It forms the backbone of any health and fitness regimen.

Now with our attached baths and crampy flats, the only way for us to get this natural gastrocolic response is with a cup of coffee / tea to 'kick start' our day. The problem according to Appa was that 'people were eating out and shitting at home, if this changed their waistline would change too,' he declared. Well modern science backs his native intelligence and like my yoga teacher Zubin sir said, scientists discover much later what an artist already knows and practises. The Stanford University has now 'researched' and 'proved' that squatting is the best position for eliminating toxins and for the health of the pelvic floor, etc. The rich, refined and educated Indian is finally gaining the confidence to squat and not sit on the pot (and is buying the squatty potty), now that it is backed by research and proved with numbers (statistics is everything). Soon they or some equally reputable institute will 'research and prove' the benefits of activity / walking before shitting too. Till then can we keep our toilets away and kitchens closer, both to our hearts and legs?

Chapter Summary

Yoga facts

- For millennia, yoga has been practised as a way of life and asanas formed an integral part of daily practice
- *Hatha Yoga Pradipika* and Patanjali's *Yoga Sutras*, are the two guiding texts summarizing yoga knowledge through the ages
- Swami Sivananda and Krishnamacharya are the two main teachers in the modern era who have carried forward the essence of yoga
- The traditional schools of yoga have been set up by the prominent students of these two teachers
- These schools of yoga more or less follow the clearly defined hierarchy or the steps of yoga practice (ashtanga) presented in the two texts
- They emphasize on yama, niyama and asana as the foundation of any yoga practice
- Only after proficiency in asana has been achieved are higher practices of pranayama and dhyana (meditation) introduced, under strict supervision
- They follow a sequence of asanas that has been fine-tuned over ages
- The sequence of asanas changes with season and the level of practice of the student, etc.
- It's important to stay light in your stomach, not empty, before performing asanas

Yoga fads

I can start a 'branch' called 'Rujuta yoga' or just 'Juta yoga' and there is nothing that you will be able to do lawfully to stop me. Or I may introduce a shoe called 'Juta yoga' and claim that it gives you a flatter stomach or a more toned butt post yoga and you will be left with no option but to BUY my product. Because **yoga belongs to our collective wisdom**, it is no one's property, at least not as yet, and even when someone can 'own' it legally in some country, it can't ethically and rightfully belong to one person or organization. And though this is in a way the acknowledgment of what our forefathers and mothers have so graciously and generously shared and refined for us, it allows for unbelievable and unmistakable malpractices. The juta yoga, for example, is a poor joke for now but can be converted into a serious business. There are many such 'businesses' or practices that very much exist out there, and below is just a broad classification:

1. Mixing yoga with some already popular exercise

For example, dance with yoga or swimming with yoga or medicine ball with yoga or aerobics with yoga or who knows, tomorrow, dumbbells and yoga.

All these forms exist with some really exotic names like moon yoga / sculpt yoga / lotus feet yoga etc., and advertise themselves as better, more logical and a greater blend of two forms of exercise or physical 'cultures'. This is exactly the problem, or to put it mildly, limitation; yoga is beyond the asana, pranayama, dhyana: it is and will remain a way of life. To reduce it to a form of 'physical culture' or 'exercise' or to 'blend' it with something is to not understand it and simply bank on the lineage and reverence it has enjoyed for centuries.

I mean you can't call some mash-up version of choreography or stretches or abdominal exercises yoga, you call them just that — dance movements or stretching or abdominal exercises. Simple enough? You may accuse me of being a purist, but it's more like if I sign up for anything 'yoga', then I want the real thing, ok?

2. Yoga in unrealistic environments

For example, hot, steamed rooms, ice slabs, mountain tops with winds blowing or unrealistic hours.

Hatha Yoga Pradipika very sternly and clearly instructs students of yoga that extremes of anything that put the body in a state of discomfort should be avoided. The very purpose of yoga practice is to go towards the true / natural state of being — which is always joyful, peaceful and harmonious. Anything which disturbs this balance and throws the physical body off gear, like practising in scorching heat / blowing winds / after cold water baths / with excessive physical strain, etc., are to be avoided.

Yoga practice should be sensible and not sensual, said BKS Iyengar at the Indo-China yoga summit, 2011, to about 1200 participants from all over the world. It would be very interesting, almost charming, to sweat profusely in a heated room or involuntary shiver on an ice slab or even to wear matching mittens and socks on a mountain top, but then it won't amount to yoga, it won't employ the intelligence of the mind, only its ability to be indulgent. **Indulgence has a name, it's called 'bhoga', and is the opposite of yoga.**

3. Yoga for specific benefits

For example, anti-wrinkle, anti-dimple, toning abs, calming the mind, seeing lights. Or for enlightenment / money / better job / sex, etc.

Hallucination is a real phenomenon and I heard a dialogue in a Harry Potter movie that went something like this: 'And what tells you that what's happening in your head is not real?' But then yoga is the ability to go beyond the argument of real and unreal. It's the art, science and above all **abhyasa of vairagya** (practice of dispassion), it's all about disowning the result and being endlessly motivated by pure practise or effort, at least that's what Patanjali's *Yoga Sutras* guides us to do. That's also what Yogeshwar (lord of yoga) Krishna said in the *Bhagwad Gita*; you are entitled to efforts only, not to its associated fruits or results. But then kya kare? Is kalyug mein, if you tell people that practise for the sake of practice, will they? Yeah! They will! And there are schools and teachers of yoga who are rude / naïve / silly / stupid / direct (choose adjective based on level of cynicism) that will teach you and tell you exactly that. The question is, are you that kind of a student? And then someone also said, when the student is ready, the teacher arrives. Till that time you can practise for the thigh gap / wrinkle-free face / lowered BP / calmer mind / enlightenment, etc., but just know that practising for benefits is always limited and not quite yoga, at least not according to Yogeshwar. Karamanevadhikaraste, remember?

4. Yoga with diet restrictions

For example, no dairy / only raw / only greens, etc.

Now I can write a book on food and yoga specifically and

demand a BIG advance by saying that it has an international market too! But see what I am thinking is already not yoga, it's planning for the future and in yoga there is now, no later, no earlier. Ya, ya, I have a long way to go and lots to learn so I won't lecture, but here goes:

Hatha Yoga Pradipika lists mitahar as one of the Yama. Yama is self-restraint (loosely put) and BKS Iyengar said at the Indo-China yoga and health summit that Yama is called 'Yama' also because that is the name of the lord of death. And for all those of you who don't follow Yama, Yama will follow you. Now, it takes a genius to put a profound philosophy so simply and with a smile. Btw, guess who was the only other speaker who was invited along with Guruji? Aha, yours truly! Hmm ... this showing off makes me more of a bhogi than a yogi, so let's get on to mitahar now.

So don't get bored and ask me why I am repeating mitahar, mitahar over and over again. You have already bought my first book and all ... but listen, back in the *Hatha Yoga Pradipika* days, both the gurus and shishya were so pahucha hua cheez that the guru would say anything only once and the shishya would abide by it for life (without the help of post-its, reminders, etc.). But even then the word mitahar and the need to abide by it gets repeated over and over in the *Hatha Yoga Pradipika*.

This is unusual and it is an acknowledgement of the fact that eating right requires daily effort, daily reminders and remains the one factor which can either propel you in the right direction or pull you back daily from the practice of yoga. Eating rice, wheat (yeah! chew that, you carb- and gluten-haters) along with herbs, spices, milk, curd, dals —

basically local, seasonal, fresh is encouraged and fasting and being drama queen with food and stale, stored, processed food is discouraged. Way before the concept of labs was even conceptualized, the yogis knew that being faddish with food would result in poor digestion, absorption, assimilation of nutrients and excretion of toxins and the practitioner would never be in a sane position to progress towards higher practices.

So that yoga farm with 'fresh' juices, quinoa khichdi and rocket leaves may be straight out of a Karan Jo fantasy but it's not yoga, and not the Yama of *Hatha Yoga Pradipika* but the other one. Get it?

Yoga FAQs

Q: *I want to learn yoga but I am worried that it goes against my religion.*

A: If anything, Yoga makes you much more religious than what you already are and enables you to absorb the essence of the religion you were born into. In Mumbai, some of the most well-known yoga gurus and strong advocates of daily asana practice are — Father Joe Pereira, a priest from Bandra Church who taught yoga to addicts in the Kripa Foundation, Shameen Akhtar who has even authored a few yoga books, Zubin Zarthotimanesh, to whom the Devi Mandir in Matunga has let out its hall permanently and from whom I currently learn.

None of them have become less Christian, Muslim or Parsi than what they were. Yoga vidya belongs to the collective wisdom of Indian sages and gurus and uplifts the life of every being who comes in contact with it, just like the sun shines as brightly whether one is rich or poor, Bahai or Jew.

Q: *I am more interested in the mental aspects than this physical circus, what yoga school should I join?*

A: Patanjali, the sage who compiled the 'best practices' across all yoga schools in India, believed that the way to progress in a sustainable manner is to follow the ashtanga in its order of hierarchy: Yama, Niyama, Asana, Pranayama, Pratyahara, Dhyana, Dharana, Samadhi.

'Until the body is put through a rigorous preparation it is in no position to control the wild elephant that is prana, the link to the bodily and mental processes.' 'Taming or controlling a wild elephant is a matter of skill, discipline.' 'A well-trained elephant could carry loads for you, an untrained one crushes you under its loads.' Metaphors like these and many more that have been passed through the oral tradition indicate that jumping straight to the 'mental processes' can be disastrous and defeat the very purpose of yoga. **The breath, much less the mind, cannot be used for the inner journey if the body hasn't learnt to stay still.** So, sorry, no shortcuts here. Asanas done correctly direct the breath and the mind to move inwards and train the senses to listen to the intelligence of both. This remains a fool-proof, time-tested and shall I say, the only way to the real union or yoga.

The best school then is the school that teaches you to be patient with the mental processes and emphasizes the importance of disciplining the body and senses first.

Q: *Isn't power yoga better than yoga?*

A: Now that depends on your definition of 'yoga', 'power'

and 'better'. I am going to assume that you mean that power yoga is some fast movements put together and better means that it will lead to you getting thinner faster. I believe it is better to have enough power in your mind to stay disciplined with your yoga practice and to be happy with the way you look. But to answer your question, a fast and vigorous movement is not power and if you read the chapter you will know what it takes to qualify as yoga. Also anything that is approached scientifically and systematically does lead to you gaining power, agility, flexibility, strength, endurance, bone density, muscle tone, etc. and reduction in body fat. And what is currently doing rounds as 'power yoga' is neither yoga nor power, it is one of those 'sweat profusely, lose weight quickly' philosophies, which I am sure by this time you have learnt to see through.

Q: *But yoga is only for flexibility na, what should I do for weight loss?*

A: Now nothing is further away from the truth. Yoga is as much about strength, endurance and cardio-respiratory fitness as it is about flexibility. It addresses all of the fitness parameters, both the aerobic and the anaerobic systems and in fact goes beyond the physical aspects of keeping you fit and lean. It has the power to give a new direction to your life altogether, you view your food differently, your body differently, you understand temptation, employ reason and begin to cherish and respect your body like never before.

Responsible behaviour with the body invariably leads to a lighter, fitter body which will eventually even lead to weight loss and tons of it. But come on, can we start appreciating life beyond weight loss?

Q: *Can I do yoga in the evening?*

A: Sure you can. Any time is a good time for yoga practice.

Q: *There is no good teacher or yoga school where I live. Can I start my practice by following books / CDs?*

A: Absolutely! That is the idea of having books. *Light on Yoga* inspired millions to practise asanas daily and it has exhaustive instructions and pictures to help you understand the how and why of every asana. There is also a book from the Bihar School of Yoga called *Asana Pranayama Mudra Bandha,* which describes asanas, and Divine Life Society sells a small booklet which teaches you how to do what they call the 12 basic postures correctly. And for beginners I like Geeta Iyengar's *Yoga in Action: A Preliminary Course* and for kids (actually even for adults) the *Yoga for Children* by Rajiv and Swati Chanchani. I believe all these books are available in bookstores or can be ordered online. I would in fact even say that if you have to choose between learning from one of these books or a teacher you are not sure about, go with the books.

Q: *Everyone in my yoga class can do the asanas much better than I can, it's demotivating.*

A: It truly is demotivating to hear that you were busy looking at other people instead of focusing on your own asanas. So first things first, watch yourself both with the inner and the outer eyes, how you feel within with every asana and how every adjustment you make in the leg, hip, back or even in your fingers and toes affects this inner experience. The purpose of yoga, after all, is to sharpen the senses to move within, the exact opposite of taking them outward and watching other people. And it helps to remember that yoga is not some competition or method to gain a smaller waist, more strength, flexibility and stamina — those are by products but not the purpose of yoga. And remember, with asanas, it's much more important to follow the right technique than reaching the final posture. The motive behind doing asanas is to progress and focus within and once you look within you will be filled with the motivation to move buildings and build bridges.

Q: *My teacher insists on doing various kriyas, etc. Should I do them?*

A: The *Hatha Yoga Pradipika* describes certain kriyas but advises extreme caution and discrimination in using them. And because hatha yoga practices are taught in an unbroken chain of guru-shisya parampara, the guru uses extreme discretion before asking you to perform any kriya, including the 'popular' kapalbhati or the 'simple' neti. My body type, for example, is not meant for any of the kriyas, so I don't do any of them nor have I been advised by any teacher to do so. BKS Iyengar says that asanas themself carry out all the purification (and more) work that is required by the body, thus eliminating the need to do kriya for 'cleansing' purposes. The kriyas are meant for therapeutic purposes and should be thought of as a therapy or drug with high potency. And just like drugs should not be bought over the counter and without prescription, similarly kriyas should not be performed just because everyone else is doing it in class. In fact, if some kriya has been prescribed for everyone in class that itself is an indication of the fact that your teacher is not using discrimination with this high-potency drug.

Q: *I do daily meditation for 1 hour. Should I continue that or start doing asanas?*

A: Meditation is not something that goes against asana practice and vice versa, both complement each other. Asanas in fact are thought of as active meditation and an essential, non-negotiable aspect of the mental preparation required to finally meditate with eyes closed. So no, you don't have to stop one to start another; asanas, if anything, will only make your meditation deeper and steadier.

Q: *What about Pilates? Isn't it just like yoga?*

A: Pilates does use some postures that are inspired from yoga but they are quite different from each other. Yoga is a philosophy of which asana practice is an integral part and is about going beyond the physical body to the annamaya kosha, and Pilates is about postures and working your core. So if you are doing Pilates, do it for Pilates and not because it is like yoga. Also, do complement it with a wholesome exercise program.

Q: *I am afraid that inversions and back bends will cause injury. And my doctor has already asked me to avoid all forward bends.*

A: Come on, first of all did you get injured doing either a back bend or an inversion? The answer, in all probability, is no. The weak back is a gift that comes with sitting around, chilling in coffee shops, getting stuck in traffic, being on con-calls etc. The inversion is a wonderful opportunity to let your spine and legs not be loaded with your body weight. The backbends make the back both stable and strong and are an essential part of the routine that is required to build a strong back and hold an erect spine. The forward bends also help you stretch the back and teach you to extend your spine. All that is required for you to do backbends, inversions, forward bends or anything under the earth safely is good technique. So asanas can teach you not just how to lengthen your spine, employ your erector spinae and strengthen your back, but also help you strengthen your legs, which not just helps prevent injuries but also teaches you a great deal about how to fall (or how to break a fall and protect the joints). So no, they won't cause injuries but will help you reduce the intensity of damage and speed up recovery should you ever get injured in the future.

Q: *Is it safe for children to do yoga?*

A: I rate TV viewing, playing of games on gadgets (however expensive) amongst the most unsafe activities for children both physiologically and psychologically. Both the mind and the body of children are malleable and asanas will ensure that they remain open and fearless in their mind, body and spirit. Asana practice is not just safe but highly recommended for young children and adolescents. One of its big advantages is that it delays and smoothens the process of puberty, extremely important in this day and age when kids seem to 'mature', lose innocence rather, at a very early age. Other than that, of course it improves their strength, flexibility, endurance and bone density. But two things are super critical here: 1. The teacher 2. The family. The teacher needs to be experienced and a serious practitioner of her art, and should have the sensibility to not teach your child 'meditation', 'pranayama', 'concentration' or any such esoteric stuff and sticks to asanas, and openly praises the child often. The family, most importantly the parents, should be practising asanas too, not because they want to encourage the child to take to yoga to improve math scores or whatever but because they believe in its philosophy and want to live by it. The book *Yoga for Children* is a good guide.

Chapter 6

Putting It All Together

As the chapter name suggests, I have tried to summarize everything we learnt in the book till now (energy systems, periodization, GAS model, FITT, etc.) into:

a) The 4 principles of exercising right
b) Real life workout recalls and their analysis.

This, I feel, will help us cross the bridge from knowing to doing, or as high funda conferences put it — from research to the field. And like the stickers behind the Mumbai rickshaws say, 'Mulgi shikli, pragati jhaali.' The girl got educated and we all progressed. The mulgi or the girl here is you, the reader. Once you learn, you progress. A rickshawalla with a funny bone wrote, 'mulgi shikli aani waat lagli', the girl got educated and screwed us all. So ya, the idea is to also screw the nonsense that goes on in the name of working out, weight loss, sculpting, wellness, etc.

a) The 4 principles of exercising right

There are 4 basic principles that every exercise program must stick to. And irrespective of your chosen form of exercise, these principles are applicable and work and most importantly, yield results. The readers of *Women & the Weight Loss Tamasha* are already aware of these but phir bhi, on public demand, here goes:

Principle 1: **Stimulate** – Do a little more every time
Principle 2: **Adap**t – The body gets used to doing what you put it through
Principle 3: **Recover** –You get fitter, stronger, leaner during recovery
Principle 4: **Regular** – Stay regular with workout, else lose out

Principle 1: Stimulate – Do a little more every time

What it means: Every workout session should be of a higher intensity than what the body is already accustomed to. This forms the mother principle of exercise — **Progressive overload principle**. So whether you choose to train the aerobic or the anaerobic, both the energy systems should be progressively overloaded. Along with them the fitness parameters of strength, endurance and flexibility should be overloaded too. But what is this 'little more'? Let's learn from the application of this principle below.

Application to your exercise:

1. Cardio – If you walk every day, do the same number of rounds of the ground and take the same time to complete them, then you are not following the Stimulate principle. Work at increasing either the number of rounds or reducing the time taken to do them. Because you must overload progressively, in one workout session do not attempt to both increase the number of rounds and decrease the time.

Here is an example of progressive overload as applied to walking:

Week 1 Week 2	Work at decreasing the time taken to cover the same distance (or same number of rounds), even if you reduce it by few seconds, it is progress. Maintain the decreased time and further reduce it by a few more seconds.	Reduce time so that RPE goes up in the range of 7-8 but never to 9
Week 3 Week 4	Work at adding ½ round without compromising on the time achieved in Week 2. Work at adding a little more distance even if it is just 10 or 20m from what you achieved in Week 3.	Increase distance so that RPE goes from 6 to 7 but never to 9
Week 5 & 6	Work at maintaining the distance achieved in Week 4 and the speed achieved in Week 2.	Maintain and practise till RPE drops to 6 and only then take it from the top.
Week 7	Take it from the top. Start the same process of Week 1 all over again and apply the same steps till the end of Week 6. Do not lose patience and rush the process, it will only lead to you wasting time, nursing injuries.	

Tip*:* The overload in a week should not be more than 10%. Though once you apply the principles, you will initially see an improvement of as much 10-15% in the first session itself, this however doesn't indicate how fit you are but only how poorly you were exercising earlier.

Calculating 10% is not always going to be easy or

practical, so you can use the RPE scale. If RPE doesn't drop in 2-4 weeks, it means that you are over-stimulated and not adapting but exhausting as a response to the stimuli.

Again by the time it's week 15 or 30, you may not be able to add more kilometres; then you can add a variation, like climbing stairs, or uphill, or change the surface from ground to sand, or sand to marsh or even the road. The point is stimulate, stimulate, expose the body to different environments.

On cardio machines the variables are: time, distance, incline or resistance, rpm or speed. So at one time, only one variable can go up, with all the others constant; remember, never more than one variable at a time. So if this week you worked on increasing the resistance, then wait until the 3rd week to increase distance.

2. Weight training – Here the variables are: set, weight and reps. At no point should all three be increased together, only one can increase at one time. Remember the point is to move in the direction of progress and not to go from 10 pounds to 100 pounds at one go. Needless to add, correct technique cannot be compromised when increasing any of these parameters.

Let's look at how you can progress:

Week 1& 2	Choose any one compound exercise for any one large muscle– e.g. squats for legs, dead lift for the back or dumbbell press for the chest and try increasing a rep for that exercise. Even if half a rep increases it is progress, alternatively work on increasing a set at the same workload, i.e. the same weight you were carrying. E.g. If you are carrying 10 lbs and doing a dumbbell press of 2 sets and 10 reps each. Either attempt to take the 10 reps to 11 or add a 3rd set. Even if you are able to push for 4 – 5 reps in the 3rd set and not to the usual 10, it is progress.	Being able to add 5 reps to your 10 reps, or ability to do full 10 reps in the 3rd set usually indicates poor exercise load to begin with.
Week 3 & 4	Work at increasing the workload or the weight you carry on the chosen exercise. So take the weight from 10 lbs to 12.5 lbs. Expect the reps to fall from 10 to a range of 6-8. If the reps fall to 3-4, then perform the rest of the 6 reps (to meet rep range of 8-10) at a lowered weight. So you can even do 2 reps at 12.5 and the rest 8 reps at 10. Do only one set at the higher weight and perform remaining sets at the same poundage, 10 in this case.	Most gyms have dumbbells separated by a 2.5 lbs, if that is not the case in your gym, ask the gym owner / management to buy more dumbbells.

Week 5 & 6 or 8	Work at maintaining all you taught your muscles from Week 1 to 4. You will see an increase in the reps of the third set along with increase in the reps of the first set where you are pushing the 12.5 lbs.	Allow your body the time to adapt and do not rush the process, even if it takes 8 or more weeks.
Week 9	Take it from the top, this time for a different muscle group. So say if Week 1 to 8 the overload was for chest, 9 to 16 can be legs, and then for the back.	

3. Yoga It is not so straightforward to apply the principle of overload to asana practice. If there is a single way to 'do more' then it is the level of penetration that you achieve in every asana, from the skin to the muscle, from the muscle to the bone, where every cell is sharp, where there is an expansion in the intellect. To quote BKS Iyengar — don't stretch your body, expand your intellect.

Tadasana can be very advance practice and mayurasana can be a beginner's practice, all depending on the approach or the refinement of the person who performs them. So this inner experience cannot be described in a book by someone like me with limited mind and limited intelligence. Asanas have the potential to take you from the limited to the unlimited, the question or the stimuli is, are you a little more tuned-in today than what you were yesterday.

Principle 2: Adapt – The body gets used to doing what it is put through

What it means: This means that the human body specifically adapts to the stimuli it experiences — in exercise science it's called **Specific adaptation to imposed demands** (SAID principle). In other words, if you work at increasing strength, then the strength will increase; if you work at increasing flexibility or endurance, then those two parameters increase respectively. Therefore it is important to stimulate every energy system, also sometimes called as principle of variation in exercise science, for overall fitness and wellbeing.

Every stimuli sets off a unique physiological, hormonal, neurological, chemical response and the body specifically adapts to it. That's exactly why running will not make you better at swimming; only swimming will make you better at swimming. This is also why a 100m sprinter cannot run a marathon: training for speed won't give your body the ability to run longer, but to run faster. And also why gymming will not give you decreased flexibility but increased strength. That's exactly why in yoga you must perform the asana on both sides, right and left, and with equal intensity. Performing an asana just on the right will bring about the benefits only on the right side. Remember how you can write only with the right hand? Even the neurological adaptation happens only on the side that has been worked out.

Application to your exercise:

1. Cardio – If you plan to run on the treadmill as your exercise today, then don't warm up on the twister or the cycle. Warm up on the treadmill only, but at a lower intensity. This allows the body to get all the required systems that the workout is going to stimulate in an alert and active position, ready to exercise.

2. Weight training – Again, treadmill or the cycle or climbing stairs will not 'warm up' the back for the dead lift, it will have to be the dead lift at a lower intensity. We have already learnt the rules of warm-up in Chapter 3.

3. Yoga – Every asana class starts with a prayer to allow you to bring the mind and the senses inwards, to allow for that expansion of the being that the asana will bring about. Vigorous stretching or flexibility exercises before the class do not serve the purpose of 'tuning in' or warming up for asanas. This is exactly why one tradition should be followed for asana practice, as the system specifically adapts and doesn't have the ability to do 'little abs, some Ashtanga and then treadmill to finish off'.

Principle 3: Recover – You get fitter, stronger, leaner during recovery

What it means: While exercise is catabolic or a breakdown in nature, it is the time after exercise, the recovery time, and what you do during that time that decides whether you will adapt to the stimuli and turn this catabolic process into an anabolic one, i.e. turn breakdown into build up.

This is where your food, drink, sleep, attitude, work-life balance, etc., come in to play. These are the real game-changers. So Santa is going through a divorce but applying the principle of 'do more' and Banta is going through courtship and applying the same principle. Who will get the chiselled look and who will get the 'I don't want to look like this' look? Kya baat hai! My sher de puttar and puttris! Well done. Banta wins and all of us win in the process. I think rest and recuperation and its effect on our entire system was beautifully depicted in the movie *Vicky Donor*. The stressed-out, urban male had poorer, weaker, slower sperm, and the chilled-out, well-rested, relaxed and easygoing boy (or rural males) had better quality and fast sperm. (Please do what Annu Kapoor does with his fingers at the word sperm.)

In weeks that you are shifting homes, offices, have guests / in-laws over, have just come back from a hectic holiday, busy with the kids' exams, preparing for your own or friend's / cousin's wedding, etc., do not bother with the principle of overload as the body will lack the required recovery to adapt to the increased stimuli.

This principle relies heavily on your commitment to eat right, the pre- and post-workout meals to carry out all the recovery and repair work. That's exactly why meal planning is an integral part of every chapter in the book.

Application to your exercise:

1. Cardio – you can perform anything the next day as the aerobic energy recovers relatively quickly. But if you have had a tough run or something and one of the TBLJ is hurting, then do some non-weight bearing cardio activity like swimming and cycling the next day. Of course, weight training can be done safely. Or you can always take the day off ☺.

2. Weight training – The anaerobic system is going to take time to recover, up to 48 hours, so no weight training back to back (even for different body parts). But you can easily put weight training and cardio on alternate days.

3. Yoga – Well, the one 'exercise' that even at the systemic, neurological, biological and across the 'pancha kosha' allows you to stimulate, adapt and never exhaust is the asana practice. Done the right way, you can practise asanas for hours daily and on all days of the week. Done the 'fast or power way', or for 'abs', 'sculpting', 'toning' purposes, limit it to 2 max 3 times a week. Actually wait, let me just be honest, just avoid it and do it zero times a week.

Principle 4: Regular – Stay regular with workout or lose out

What it means: Le mar! The place where all science will come to a grinding halt and only discipline will see you through is right here, right now. Regularity doesn't mean daily but only means keeping your date with your workout (even if it's once a week) and no matter what, not pushing it to tomorrow, evening or next week, etc.

See, if you have a well-functioning mind, it is always going to give you 100 options in 100 milliseconds to the prospect of working out. But if you have a well-functioning intellect, it will have the discriminating ability to understand the mind and to know that if one of those 100 options is used, then at the next prospect of exercise, 1000 options will be offered.

The way forward is to carry out the exercise exactly when planned and to know that once the exercise begins the mind goes silent and bows down to the intellect. This is easier said than done, and that's exactly why Patanjali's *Yoga Sutra* says that if you have to choose between *vairagya* and *abhyasa*, abhyasa is more crucial. In our world of attachments, vairagya is probably impossible but with enough abhyasa, discipline, we can reach the state where the workout itself provides the entire fulfilment and joy and not the associated weight loss.

Application to your exercise:
Cardio, weight training or yoga, each one is tough, the mind does imagine hurdles: oh! I have to wear certain shoes, the tights I want are in the machine, I am not going to get parking, this is when all treadmills will be full. But know that just moving in the direction of your door and out of the house works like magic over these perceived problems. And once you begin exercising there is that blessing of the BDNF loop, the feel good, the high, the worthiness and the boost of self-esteem. So just go for it meri jaan.

Chalo, the other side of the story is the use it or lose it funda (yes it makes an appearance once again). If you do not provide your body with the stimuli of exercise then it is going to reverse all that you gained with exercise over months and years, the sweat and blood — that taut face, the flat stomach, the speed, the agility, the strength, the stamina, the hormones — in as little as 2 to 8 weeks (called as the principle of reversibility). But like a ray of hope, it will give you the muscle memory, so stop crying and start moving.

Home fitness tests

Fitness assessment is a major tool that I use while assessing the progress of my clients. The equation is very simple, if they are doing well on the tests then their body composition is improving, and so are all metabolic parameters — thyroid, insulin sensitivity, BP etc. And because the tests compare you to you, they give you a much more real picture as against comparing you to some 'standard'.

Some of the most common fitness tests are:

a) *Sit and reach test to measure your flexibility*
b) *Core strength and stability test to measure the strength in the muscles*
c) *VO_2 max test to measure your aerobic fitness*

You can ask your trainer to conduct a fitness assessment test for you or you can check out www.exrx.net and learn to do it yourself.

All of the above are home fitness tests, something which you can do easily without the intervention of an expert, equipment or costs. These tests have been designed by sport coaches to basically give us an idea of the direction we are moving in. These are not meant to depress you, or to be cracked by cheating. Assess your fitness every 12 weeks. Before every test, warm up adequately, stretch and only then begin the test. And yes, please don't perform the test empty stomach, eat a fruit or a little something, you know the rules of pre-workout meals now.

b) Real life workout recalls and analysis

Truth is stranger than fiction. Nowhere is this more valid than what happens in the real world of diets and workouts. I had put diet recalls of some of my clients in the earlier two books, but of late it's the workout recalls that have often stumped me with their sheer 'wow' factor. I mean, even if I try my best I can't make these up.

My clients accuse me of being an autocrat because I get them to write their workout recalls along with the diet recall. 'Why write? I know I am doing it all wrong, just tell me what to do.' 'But how do I tell you what to do without knowing what you do? Spend a week writing and that in effect will save us a lot of time,' I goad them. They give in and send me their weekly workout recalls. Sharing some with you along with how and why the workout plans were changed, and hoping that this will help you spot mistakes in your own and make corrections.

For quick reference, following are the situations / workouts / personalities covered in detail below:

1. Overtraining
2. Cardio to lose the paunch
3. Punishing legs for being fat
4. No recovery / just walking
5. The 'kill the bitches' workout
6. The monk with the Ferrari
7. The player

1. Overtraining

I was working with a very dedicated 20-something doctor, who lived in a hostel and was in that crucial stage of life — doing rounds with senior doctors and generally feeling super overwhelmed with what all a doctor is supposed to do and not do and with the attitude they have to build to survive and thrive. It's also the stage where you just follow a senior doc like a sheep and are generally treated badly by both patients and the doctor; 'it's like a slug fest,' she said. 'All this I can take easily,' she admitted, but it's the cousin's wedding where she wanted to metamorphose like Deepika of *Yeh Jawaani Hai Diwani*, from chashmish to charming. 'Hmm. You are already so charming,' I said and it was really heartfelt. She was amongst my stars. Rasika had got herself an electric cooker and a plate and had started cooking dal-rice in the dingy hostel room. I mean she did everything that I asked of her and so diligently. Then I also asked her to incorporate weight training into her routine, just 2 days a week and she did. But then she wrote me a long email about how that made her feel dizzy and sleepy on rounds and that was just not acceptable. 'Write down all you do in the gym,' I said and so she did and this is what we found:

The original workout recall:

Day 1	*1 n half hour of cardio ie 20 min tread mill, 15 min cycle, 15 min cross trainer, floor exercises twister n sides*
Day 2	*1 hour of wt training and 15 min of treadmill and 15 min of cycle*
Day 3	*same cardio for 1 n half hour*
Day 4	*missed gym so did aerobic dance for 15 min, biceps n shoulders without dumbless, a total of 20-25 min*
Day 5	*wt training for 1 hour and tread mill for 25 min and twisting for 2-3 min*
Day 6	*rchd home wanen to workout but felt very dizzy so jus 10 min of tread mill n I stopped*
Day 7	*same thing again I went to gym but was dizzy. So jus did 10 min of cycle n 5-7 min of treadmill but cudnt do…*

Analysis:

Now unlike most people I work with, an intern doc is

physically active, walking around quite a bit during the day, sometimes at a length for about 6-8 hours. Just a glance at her recall and you know that Rasika is a victim of overtraining. 'But the more calories I burn, the more I lose,' was her logic.

The 1½ hour of cardio with floor and twisters thrown in is in no way going to burn fat but will just put her in a hypoglycaemic state.

And doing cardio post weight training for an hour only meant staying in the catabolic zone, wasting muscle tissue, delaying both adaptation and recovery from the workout.

Then she did that cardio and twisting all over again.

The aerobic dance at home was not out of joy but the guilt of missing the gym, that itself renders it as a useless activity and not a fat-burning one. And curling your arms or raising them over the head without dumbbells to a point of exhaustion, is not strength training, it is stupidity.

After that, with double josh and double guilt of 'missing gym yday', madam worked out, but again that long cardio post weight training put the body in the punishment zone. Wasting the hard-earned lean tissue, bringing the fat-burning to a halt and leading to poor recovery from stimuli. Rasika had entered the over-trained, exhausted stage.

Thankfully, because her body had developed intelligence through eating right and because the body always prioritizes survival over 'fat burning', it went into damage control mode, very kindly felt dizzy, and ensured that further muscle wastage was prevented. This 'feeling dizzy couldn't gym', also allowed for much-needed recovery time. This is how Rasika's workout was reworked:

Modified workout plan:

Day 1	Run and walk	30 mins RPE 6-7
Day 2	Week by week sequence from Iyengar Yoga beginners guide.	We had two reasons for this – 1. To learn inversions – we need to balance work and family life without feeling that we are losing out on either (girls want it all) so the inversions keep our strength and hormones in a good place. And all that mental activity that her job put her through meant we had to work on providing more oxygen and blood to the over worked brain. 2. Cellulite – the precision of asanas that the Iyengar style teaches helps you rid the body of the ugly orange peel – because it teaches you how to reach deep within and employ the unused muscle tissue lying under layers of fat.
Day 3	Upper body strength training	Sample 2-day split from strength training chapter
Day 4	Cardio	45 mins RPE 6-7 And because she so loved doing abs, she did two sets of regular crunches before the cardio (not after, better use of glycogen).
Day 5	Rest	

Day 6	Lower body strength training	We sandwiched legs workout between two days of rest because her current assignment had a lot of walking already. The rest day before legs was to ensure that she got a chance to replenish as much glycogen as she could so that legs could get a chance to train under a full tank.
Day 7	Rest	The next day was rest too, as she had very little scope to actually rest the legs given her walking around in the hospital. But with those 24 hours of full recovery she could walk and not drag herself on sore legs at the work place.

Over a period of time she learnt to do the restorative postures for accelerating recovery not just in the gym but in the hospital too. And yeah, she even danced at the wedding to *Dilli Wali Girlfriend*, just for cheap thrills ;).

2. Cardio to lose the paunch

Feroze is a 33-year-old ad executive. He is a hardworking guy and joined the gym when he changed jobs. His earlier job had got him fat and his aunt told him that Nashira should get a new husband now that he looked more like her dad than husband. And he complained that overall he was fine, just his paunch, he needed to lose his paunch, baaki his face and all was Mashallah! ;)

After much begging at his lotus feet, he sent me a scanned copy of his workout recall. It is a pure 'lose that paunch workout', he added.

Original workout recall:

Day 1 :- 45 mins Cardio — 300 Cals
ABBS :- 4 Variation 3 sets 20 Reps
Waist : 3 " " "

Day 2 : 20 mins EFX :- 100 Cals
Upper Body :- 2 Variation 20 Reps
Low Back :- 2 Variation 25 Reps.

Day 3 :- 40 mins Cardio — 250 Cals
Legs :- 6 Variation 20 Reps
All with Body Weight.

Burns 50 Calorie on treadmill in 10 mins

Burns 105 Carlorie on EFX in 10 mins

Lifts upto 3 kg Dumbell.

He then repeats the same on day 4, 5 and 6.

Analysis:

Since you understand how EEE is calculated, this 'burned 300 cals or 100 cals in 10 mins, etc.,' will no longer interest you. 'What about after-burn Feroze,' you will ask. 'Baba EPOC kidhar hai?' See I can read your mind, and that is going to be my next profession if you throw me out of my current line of work. With those 4 and 3 variations each for abs and waist, amounting to 20 reps each, what is Feroze burning — fat or time? Shall we rename this book as, don't burn your cash, burn your fat?

Now resting metabolism, i.e. when Feroze is driving, sitting in meetings, lounging on the sofa and channel surfing, is predominantly aerobic metabolism and can therefore 'theoretically' burn fat. But without the after-burn effect, he won't burn more fat than what he is currently burning at rest, and soon that mashallah face will start developing a double chin!

Also he is dedicating much more time and sets to his abs and waist than his entire upper and lower body. In fact, with that paunch and all that jarring that the spine will go through with his variations of abs and waist, the lower back will be at a huge risk of developing symptoms ranging from mild weakness and stiffness to a full-blown slip disc. Not to forget the independent risk factor of sitting, which Feroze does most of the time. Also on the days he trains his legs, he has already done cardio for 45 minutes, so there go our glycogen stores. No wonder then, that he lifts no weight and does some 6 variations of exercises only on 'body weight': he has no fuel (glycogen) left to actually channelize his anaerobic energy.

And what is this 'lifts 3 kg dumbbells'? Are you SRK, Feroze? Why are you referring to yourself in third person? 'Arre meri ma! That's coz I can't relate to myself in the gym, I'd rather play cricket, but no one will take me in their team and I don't have money to join fancy clubs. Plus I don't like all this pumping-shumping, but if I run or walk outside, I sweat so much that I have to take a bath before going to the office and generally it's a lot of wasted time ya.'

Modified workout plan:

Anyway, keeping in mind all of Feroze's problems of time and embarrassment at being in the gym (the people and bulky trainers were 'so intimidating', and he hated the music they played too), we devised a training plan.

Day 1	Walk/jog on sand	30-40 mins RPE – 6-7 Kept this on Sunday as that was holiday so enough time for bathing, etc.
Day 2	Rest OR Suryanamaskar 2 rounds	Learnt Sivananda style suryanamaskar from the same aunt who wanted Nashira to get a new husband ☺
Day 3	Upper body strength training	Cost him about 30 mins and didn't break into too much of a sweat so quick shower and change in the gym and off to office.
Day 4	Rest	
Day 5	Lower body strength training	From the 2-day split plan as in the sample workout. Legs are always the biggest calorie burner and the real 'lose the paunch' agents.
Day 6	Rest	
Day 7	Climbed stairs in the building	Began with climbing 6 floors (RPE at 7-8) at a time. Climbed up and came down by lift. The goal was to climb higher and higher in the same 20 mins. This trained him in the anaerobic zone and the Day 1 training used all the lactic acid he produced for generating ATP aerobically. Well atleast that's how we planned it on paper ;).

3. Punishing legs for being fat

Jinal is your typical housewife, all of 38, with grown-up kids who no longer need constant attention except during exams of course. She passes her time by investing heavily in shares and raking in heavy profits. 'Whatever the economy, you feel it in your stomach, when to enter and when to exit, and it is so much fun,' is her take on it. She lives with her in-laws and also cooks, cleans, supervises and takes active part in household 'duties'. Her big fear is that she would look like her mom and mom-in-law: huge on her thighs, right under the butt. 'My waist is small, arms are ok too, but the sides, the "saddle bags", are stubborn.'

'I do lot of cardio but this,' pinching the sides of her thighs, 'is not going. Can your diet help me cut it and throw it in the Arabian sea?' 'Just start weight training,' I said with a straight face. 'The more muscle fibres you recruit, the more after-burn you will have post exercise. So while you play money-money, fat will burn at a higher rate honey-honey ;).'

'Get a good trainer from your gym, sign up for personal training atleast for few sessions.' But money is not something she liked to spend, especially on training and all that. Anyway, she told me that first she would like to get regular and only after that would she think of a personal trainer; till then, she said, 'I will manage'. 'Ok, write what you do, that way I know that you are not mismanaging anything.' So she filled up the exercise tracker sheet we sent her and this is how it read:

Original workout recall:
Exercise Tracker

Date	*Exercise*	*Sets*	*Weights (Lbs/Kgs)*	*Repetitions*
29th Aug	*Leg Press/ Leg Curl/ Leg Extension Adductor/ Abductor Dumbell Press Seated Rows Push ups/ Dumbbell Curl*	*2 2 2 2 2 2 2 2*	*20/ 40 lbs/ 40 lbs/ 25kgs 20/25 lbs 5 /10 lbs 40 lbs 40 lbs*	*20 20 20 20 20 20 20 20*
31st Aug	*Leg side kick (pyramid set)/ Leg Curl / Seated leg press (super set) Leg kick back (in glute machine) Lying leg press/ leg ext/calf raise (super set)*	*3 / 3 / 3*	*50lbs /80lbs /30lbs*	*15*
On all other days I go for a walk or walk on treadmill at very high speed and incline.				

Analysis:
Jinal ben is going all out to punish her legs for getting fat. She has devised a workout with the help of some friends who had the 'same problem' and had merged that with the cut-outs of

'get that butt', 'shake it like Shakira', 'Squeeze, not sorry' and 'burn the flab', etc., from her collection of various women and fashion magazines.

Now her strength training plan only focuses on her legs and completely behaves like she may not have a back, chest, shoulders, arms, etc. There are just some random exercises for the upper body. The second day in the gym is also 'dedicated' to legs with the 'super set' she learnt from the 'Shake it like Shakira' article.

On Day 1 of weight training, leg press is the only compound exercise she has done, which has employed multiple joints and multiple muscles and on that she has lifted the least amount of weight because she doesn't want to 'bulk up'. Then on extensions, curls, adductors, abductors, she goes all out and pushes either as much or double of what she has pushed on the leg press as that is where she wants to 'burn' it all from. Also the rep range is 20, because again, the fashion mag informed her that high reps and low weight is for fat burning. Of course fashion mags and tabloid columns don't have the patience for EPOC and don't really care about how much fat you may burn from exercise and other such factors.

When it comes to the upper body, she barely lifts any weight with the back, but with the bicep, which is only an assisting muscle, she lifts as much as 40 pounds! The chest gets a decent workout but is not in proportion to the back and hence even if the chest responds, she is going to have an awkward upper body appearance.

The second day in the gym she uses 'super sets', where she trains 3 main movements, or exercises, back-to-back without a break and hopes for reduction in size from 'target area', just as the gossip columns promised. Now super sets, pyramid sets, drop sets are very advanced methods of training, best employed by body builders or people who are decently strong and can squat under a bar that weighs at least as much as they do. So if you are 50 kg and can squat for about 8 reps under a bar of 50 kg, then by all means go super set, drop set, do whatever you want and the body will respond. But when you have only just about begun training, keep the focus on learning the technique, be strict with your form, stay consistent with your gym schedule, plan your post-workout meals, basically stay safe, workout with efficiency and make recovery (adaptation to training) a priority.

Let's look at her cardio — very high speed and incline, when someone says that, I picture a person holding the rails of the treadmill, leaning backwards and turning the neck to see how flabby the thighs look as they pop up and down with every step. Ah! Just the imagination hurts both my back and my brain, so go with this thumb rule: when on incline, the speed should be easy; when the speed is high, incline should be zero. At any point of time only one variant or component of training should change / challenge; never more than one. So in cardio, if time goes up, reduce intensity. If speed goes up, reduce time.

Anyway, the way she is training has to change because it's her muscle fibre recruitment that is going to decide the amount of calories she will burn during and after and also influence how strong she gets. Only strong thighs don't look flabby.

Modified workout plan:

Day 1	Lower body in the gym	From the 2-day split plan. To optimize muscle fibre recruitment to gain more tone and bone mineral density in the legs.
Day 2	Rest / easy walk on the treadmill or grass	Just to keep her active and to go easy on the joints.
Day 3	Spinning class in the gym	Cycling is a non-weight bearing activity.
Day 4	Upper body in gym	To ensure proportionality in upper and lower body.
Day 5	Treadmill or walk 40 mins with intermittent jog.	Got her off the incline but added the jog to help her feel that she is 'sweating it out'.
Day 6	Rest	
Day 7	Day with the kids at the park	Free play – active interaction outside of studies;) Also sent a strong message that play is as important as school (if not more).

'Solid returns on low investment,' Jinal said when she described the 'saddle bags' to me on the phone within 4 weeks of the program. 'But how when I am not doing a single adductor / abductor? But don't tell me, I don't even want to know. Mere se zyaada my husband is happy, uska stress khatam ho gaya because I no longer ask him whether I look fat on the thighs. Nahi toh, you know na, every answer is wrong, ha bolega toh bhi maraa and nahi bolega toh bhi.' The husband shouted out a 'thanks Rujuben' in the background.

4. No recovery / Just walking

Mrs Kapadia, a matriarch with a huge mansion, lawns and a very happy family with caring sons and daughters-in-law had exactly one problem in life: kambakht weight! And with that of course there was 'knee problem'. 'Nothing serious right now,' her doctor informed her. 'Just lose 15 kg and you will be fine.'

Very promptly then, one of the daughters-in-law shared her personal trainer with my client and this is what she started doing:

Original workout recall: *(From her trainer's email to me)*

Here is madam's workout schedule:

1. *Normal walk in the park for 30 minutes — 3 days a week*
2. *One hour workout with trainer — 3 days a week*

The breakdown as follows.

a. *30 minutes treadmill — level speed 5 to 6. incline level 2 once in a few days.*

the next 30 minutes is distributed as:

b. *50 times throw ball — hold with both the hands*
c. *cable pull up + upper body exercise + alternate weight or boxing*

Analysis:

Obviously Mrs Kapadia can change a lot of things in here. Is she working out? Yes, religiously walking every day for 30 minutes and every alternate day doing some 'toning' or 'light training' all in the hope of losing weight and making the knee feel better.

But one look and you can see that there is no strength training for the legs at all. When I asked her why, she said, 'But I am already walking for the lower body and I don't want to overdo on a weak knee.' Well, you see, with all that walking, the weak knee is going to get weaker and its weakness is going to be compounded by the fact that there is just no strength training in there for the legs. The strength in the legs will go up only if there is that specific stimuli for the leg muscles, tendons, bones and ligaments, and that will come with the usual suspects: leg press, squats, lunges, extensions, curls, etc.

Also, the upper body will need much more than just throwing a ball, cable pull-up and some 'upper body exercises'. We will still need to follow the big muscles before small muscles, compound before single joint and the whole sequence we learnt in strength training. And because you read the cardio chapter well too, if Mrs Kapadia is already having 'knee problem', which means that the TBLJ and muscles are weak, should she be walking every day? And between treadmill and walk in the park, i.e. grass, what surface should she choose? Also, while the knee is weak, does it make sense to walk on an incline? Wow! Thank you God! For blessing me with earnest and intelligent readers ☺.

Modified workout plan:

So let's apply what we know and plan her workout. The first thing that we should plan for her is REST, because without adequate recovery, the body will never adapt and instead reach the exhaustion stage, our dreaded phullishestop! So here goes:

Day 1	Rest	
Day 2	Walk in the park – chose grass or mud path	Steady state – walk at a speed that can be maintained easily for 30mins. RPE of 4-5
Day 3	Strength training for full body	Till the legs don't gain enough strength it's foolish to stimulate them with too many sets or keep a separate training day for them. They have to be stimulated with patience and given enough time to recover and adapt from the stimuli.
Day 4	Rest	But walking around at home is encouraged.
Day 5	Cycle on a stationary bike	Work at covering more distance today and limit it to 20 mins. RPE of 5-6
Day 6	Iyengar yoga therapy class	Helped her with pelvic opening, strengthening of the quads, flexibility of the hamstrings and strength in the butt.
Day 7	Walk on treadmill	For 20-30 mins (because she liked the treadmill, plus her son specially got it for her so she didn't want to waste money now). RPE of 4-5

This is what we began with, and in 8 weeks she looked better, thinner and the knee pain had disappeared. 'How is it possible?' she asked me. 'I have hardly lost any weight (must have been about 3 to 4 kg) and I hardly work out.' Now if the body composition changes, the muscles begin to hypertrophy, the TBLJ feel the love and don't get jarred daily and once the fat mass begins to recede then knee pain toh jayega na? And don't forget the brain's analgesic effect in response to exercise.

5. The 'kill the bitches' workout

'I am doing a faadu workout and no one, no one in my gym can do what I do,' boasted Neelima. 'Good!' I said. 'Kya fayda? I am not thin, see this.' She stood up and picked up the roll of fat that covered the button on top of the jeans. 'Like diet se farak pada hai, I can do more exercise and I look thinner but not as thin as I want. After my workout, I can't even walk out of the gym, I want someone to carry me out. Matlab I walk out but I am like a zombie. You watch *The Walking Dead*? Something like that. Wanting someone to shoot me in the head so that I can die instead of living with my fat, my jiggly thighs, aching knees and freaky arms.' 'Please stop describing yourself like that! Your body can hear you. Just send me your workout routine.' And this is what came in.

Original workout recall:

Day 1 – Cardio workout

10 workouts, each 3 mins with 20 sec in between

Warm up + stretching (5 mins)

1. *Jogging*
2. *cycling*

3. *bench jumps (plyometrics)*
4. *Stepper*
5. *Ski machine*
6. *Jump over step bench*
7. *Row machine*
8. *Jog with 10 kg bag*
9. *Squats on ball*
10. *Step jump (10 reps) with push-ups (10 reps)*
11. *Cool down (5 mins)*

Day 2 – Full body workout called 'Belts, bands, Bajao!' (because we use only bands, balls, TRX and work out till we die) OR Functional workout

Warm up (10 mins)

Each of the following sets lasts 40 sec each with 20 sec break in between

1. *Squats + single-legged squats (2 sets)*
2. *Low row (2 sets)*
3. *Chest press (2 sets)*
4. *Tricep extensions (2 sets)*
5. *Bicep curls (sets)*
6. *Suspension lunges (3 sets)*
7. *Hamstring curls (2 sets)*
8. *Plank Crunch (2 sets)*
9. *Suspended lateral Plyo-push up (2 sets)*
10. *Pike Crunch (2 sets)*
11. *Cool down (5 mins)*

Day 3 – Fitness Challengers

Warm up + stretching (10 mins)

All workouts below performed 3 sets (21 reps, 15 reps, 9 reps) with 30 sec break between workouts. No break between sets. below workout done with 2 nos. 5 kg plates

1. *Incline push ups with both feet on the step bench + combination barbell shoulder press & squatting on the way down*
2. *(lying on the step-up) barbell pullover with tricep raises combination workout + squat jumps*
3. *mountain climber + combination of barbell front raise & barbell upright row*
4. *rear barbell + ski jumps using step bench (alternating between left and right leg while maintaining the squat position)*
5. *squats while holding plate (5 kg) upright + ab crunch with 5 kg plate*

This is a 3-day split and it is then repeated so that way I am working out 6 days a week. My trainer is kickass man and I am secretly in love with his sweaty, smelly armpits. His mouth stinks but he eats chewing gum all day. I find this both practical and sexy but also annoying. I don't know why I am telling you all this, but you know everything anyway about my life so no problem, just don't use it in some book or blog. Actually use it, who bloody cares!

Analysis:

Now I know what you're thinking, I have the most amazing job in the world, and I will confirm that it really is. Won't trade these kind of moments for anything. But seriously, being drawn, very strongly, to your trainer is not unusual. Like some scriptwriter, they belong to a world of their own where only muscles live and fat dies, like actors they stare at themselves in the mirror while training you so you never get the chance to feel conscious about you staring at them, like fools they understand nothing about money, economy, history, world politics, and all this adds to their raw appeal. So stare at them, fall in love with them, but still only train, don't strain with them.

For starters, this is not a '3-day split', it is gym jargon used for 3 'kill the bitches' sessions. Ya, that's what you guys and gals are called when you keep telling your trainers 'but I am not losing only'. Physical exertion and exercise are poles apart. You can exert yourself while carrying your baby in the mall, running across Andheri station to get to Churchgate fast, etc., but then just because you did it 3 times, with a 20 second break in between, it won't qualify as exercise, much less lead to any fat burning, your ultimate goal in life.

Anyway let's look at Day 1. 'It's a circuit training in cardio and you are just jumping from one station to another. Gosh! But that's all you do on all days. So you will need at least one steady state cardio, where you teach your body to sustain an activity for about 30 to 45 minutes. Also, when your knees are not very happy with the current weight that is falling on them why jog with a sack of 10 kg and jar your joints? And you are doing the squats on a ball to protect your knees, when actually squats even under a bar of 10 kg will be so much easier on your knees than that jog.' 'Maybe because I am already putting stress on my knees with the jog, my trainer wants to ease it out for me with squats on the ball.' Ok, exercise science loses, smelly underarms win.

'The next day again, bands, balls, tubes and suspension wires — are you shooting some action sequence for *Dhoom 3*? Remember the GAS model — Stimulate, adapt and don't exhaust? And I think you actually have the strength to do a proper 3-day split where you can train legs, chest-shoulder-tricep and back-biceps on 3 different days. Why are you mixing all muscles in random order on one day; there is no stimuli here to adapt, this will just exhaust. You know if the strength in your quads went up even by as little as 20% (which is a very reasonable expectation out of a well-structured strength training plan) then this whole knee pain can disappear?' 'No, but you know this is army work out, the US army also does this in Afghanistan.' 'Yes but they do this whole belts, bands, ball thing because there are no gyms there, and remember they are super fit to begin with, so this won't exhaust them but it will exhaust you.' 'Ha, even I am doing this for fitness only; from next time we are doing this with jumps on tyres.' Ok, smelly underarms win again.

'Also the fitness challengers day is actually muscle confusion theory, this time we did this but next time my trainer will come up with something else, so we never know what to expect.' 'Listen, only we are confused here, the muscles are not. The only "confusion" or surprise they need is the progressive overload principle, where they learn to contract under forces that are higher than the ones normally encountered. There is no "confusion" to be achieved with random mixing of exercises. In fact, for optimal fat burning, the sequence of big muscles before small muscles, compound before isolation, warm up specificity, etc., must be followed. Also if you remember your exercise science, while going from 21 reps to 9 reps you actually go from aerobic to anaerobic but you are not able to lift higher weight on 9 reps as compared to what you lift on 21 reps because of the low glycogen status.

If you let your body train under what it can actually lift for 9 reps with good technique, you would be lifting much more than 5 kg. That's when you get the after-burn. In all you are not training, simply straining.'

Modified workout plan:

Finally we did mandavli, I never wanted her to lose sight of the gum-chewing, smelly-armpits trainer because it was he who was responsible for her rapchik exercise compliance, even at the cost of her aching knees and cramping calves, so this is what we came up with:

Day 1	25m sprints	6 times with 1 min walk in between.
Day 2	40 mins jog	On a soft surface, for her it was on the beach.
Day 3	Lower body strength training	Cost her about 45 mins to an hour. Worked on increasing her strength in quads, hips, calves, hams and legs are always the big calorie burners ;).
Day 4	Stretching class	Thankfully her trainer conducted a stretching class too, which madam earlier didn't go to because 'it was not for burning calories'.

Day 5	Any one of the 3 workouts which she 'loved' and didn't want to give up on	Ideally would have liked to see her on one of the cardio machines, either the elliptical or cycle, to reduce the load / impact on the knees.
Day 6	Upper body strength training	Upper body strength is crucial because once the knee aches, the hip, lower back, upper back, neck all begin to overcompensate or feel the strain. It's important to protect all joints, not just the aching ones.
Day 7	Rest	Thankfully one rest day

'Look, how tight my abs have become,' she said while getting me to touch her midriff. 'Wow!' I exclaimed. 'Even my trainer tells everyone now that I am his star, he gives everyone my example and says, train like her. Train, don't strain!' My sister would call this 'win-win'. Science finally wins along with the sweat and smell of hairy underarms ;).

6. The monk who has not sold his Ferrari

Shyam babu led the life of a yogi with the Ferrari. And like most of my clients, he advised, mentored and held a mirror for me. 'You are wasting your time,' he informed me. According to him, any business that is not worth a minimum of 200 crore rupees is a pure waste of time, and all this 'keeping up quality and not spreading out' is purely my inefficiency. He only believed in yoga and no other form of 'artificial' exercise. One 'sir' came home every morning at 4 a.m. because 'that is the Bramhamahurata, the ideal time for practice', and from 4-6 a.m. Shyam babu and sir practised yoga. Shyam babu's yoga practice and business skill was legendary in Kanpur business circles and from the day he had started, he hadn't skipped even a day.

However, his BP wouldn't budge and he couldn't fathom why. He was doing everything; every asana that would 'benefit' heart, gas, cholesterol, etc., was in the routine, so was a glass of 'drinks' every night for 'relax'. He came to me for his diet because 'book thodi spiritual type lagi' and he thought Skype was a good way to meet, no need to fly to Mumbai from Lucknow. His diet was already really good, local and seasonal and the wife and staff at home were devoted, bringing his dabbas to office and cooking exactly as he liked; no one really would want to get on his wrong side.

'Your diet is good, you love your work, your family life is in harmony, there's no reason why BP, cholesterol and constipation should affect you,' I said to him. And this man was disciplined; not skipping a 2-hour daily practice for over 6 years is no easy task. 'So what kind of yoga do you really do?' 'Patanjali yoga,' he answered. 'All yoga is Patanjali yoga, Shyam babu. What school is your sir from?' 'What do you mean what school?' 'I mean, what tradition does he follow?' 'Ha! Woh sab ka mix — thoda Bihar school, thoda Iyengar, thoda Patanjali par ab aap kehte ho ke sab Patanjali hai? Aur thoda weight loss, 15-20 suryanamaskar, pranayama, meditation, ekdum all round program banaya hai humne.' 'Abhi mera dimaag bhi pura all round ho gaya, aap likheye na please, then we will know exactly what you are doing,' I asked him. He did, and this is what it read like:

Original workout recall:

Group 1 *SURYA NAMASKAR -12* *Core Work - single leg up, then opposite side, up again then down to 20 deg - 10 on each leg* *Did the same with two legs* *Cycling* *Bending and straightening* *Open the leg wide at 90 deg and closing* *Leg up to 90 Deg - in 8 counts, dropping the leg to 20 Deg* *Rolling and Rocking* *Utkat asan with wall (Had the block bet the thigh)* *Utkat asan on the mat* *Garur asan with the wall* *Garur Asan on the mat* *Warrior 2* *Pashvakon* *Pashvoveer* *Warrior 1* *Wide angle forward bend and then into side lunging* *Wide angle forward bend to lunge by taking the right arm under the leg - Both sides* *Knelt down and then extend one leg and then side stretching (Gate Pose)* *Pigeon* *Wide angle chakki* *Wide angle boat rowing* *Squatting and wood Chopping* *Squat and then forward bend* *Kapal Bhati (3 sequence of 100 each)*	*Group 2* *Tadasan* *Triyaka Tadasan* *Kati Chakra* *Single leg lift and then double leg lifts* *Single circles and then double* *Single leg cycling and then double leg cycling* *Knees circle* *Spinal twists* *Rolls & Rocks* *Navasan* *Sit with leg stretch and do shakti bandha including chakki and boat rowing with legs together and legs apart* *Squat* *Wood chopping* *Twisting* *Crow walking and then back* *Squat forward bending* *Classical surya Namaskar 12* *Anuloma – Viloam – 10 rounds`* *Nadi shodhan – 10 rounds* *Om meditation – 10 rounds* *End with Savasana.*

'This is your weekly routine?' 'Daily,' he answered. 'Har subaha 4-6 a.m., itna accha program ban gaya hai, now everyone wants to work out with my trainer, ekdum in demand he has become. Just like you after Kareena, nahi toh pehle aap ko kaun puchta tha?' 'You do this daily?' I was still stuck on that. 'Yes, don't even miss a Sunday.' 'Don't you get tired?' 'Nahi nahi, aaram se karta hu up to 6 o'clock, then I do savasana, then 9-9.30 breakfast.' 'And in between?' 'Savasana! I do savaasana till 8-8.30.'

Analysis:
Wohoo... I was about to pass into unconsciousasana! Your trainer may be famous in Kanpur, Kandivali, Kanyakumari or Kashmir, but famous and expensive doesn't always convert into efficient, safe and practical! Boy! Who does 'savasana' for 2 hours? It's more like slipping into hypoglycaemia post movements that are parading themselves as 'yoga'.

First things first — is doing yoga as the only form of exercise enough? It's more than enough even to live by. And will it give you weight loss? Of course it will, but you have got to pursue it with 'abhyasa' and 'vairagya', just like the way Patanjali asked you to. That's with in-depth understanding, practice, perseverance, patience and non-attachment to its 'weight losing', 'relaxing', 'gas nikaling', 'stomach losing' benefits. And it's best to stick to a teacher who belongs to and believes firmly in one tradition / school of yoga. All traditions eventually meet at the same destination and are meant to cater to people of different temperaments, and each tradition continues to draw and inspire from the other, but will never give up on its core to be like the other.

Following one tradition means following a ritual of practice that is safe, a sequence that is well thought out from beginning to end, is a sensible and not a sensuous practice. The minute you have a teacher who is mixing everything, you have a half-baked person who is himself confused and unsure about what will work, and how it works. Someone who is willing to reduce yoga practice to vigorous movements: sometimes with the limbs, at other times, very stupidly and dangerously, with the breath. Together this is a deadly combo, it may not kill you immediately but it will lead to a more confused state of both the mind and body, in fact your whole being.

The Bihar School of Yoga teaches you a primary, intermediate and advanced group of asanas. The Ashtanga (Mysore) style calls it the series. The Sivananda school focuses on 12 postures and introduces new ones based on the practise of the students. The Iyengar school lists out asana routines on a day-by-day basis and tells you how to progress your practise into weeks, months and years. Each one of them has a complete practice which needs no tweaking, much less mixing from new age yoga teachers or gurus. Having said that, it is not uncommon for yoga teachers and students to follow different classical traditions for different needs: for example, Iyengar yoga for asana practice and learning music from the Agra gharana along with Vedic studies from Swami Parathasarthy or Rakeshbhai or Dada because all these different activities also find their roots in the yoga philosophy. So this kind of a mix is ok, the other kind is not, ok? By the other kind I mean trikonasana from Iyengar, kapalbhati from the camp you attended in office and the thigh busting postures your cousin taught you on a trip to Mussourie, all rolled into a 1 hour yoga practice is not ok. Not ok. Not ok. Not ok. Ok?

Modifications:

After an equally passionate and anger-filled lecture, Shyam babu agreed to follow the *Beginners Guide to Yoga* by BKS Iyengar which we had sent him, so that he could learn how to do his poses and do them in the correct sequence. He followed that religiously too, but this time, the gas, cholesterol and BP came down too. 'So much better in just 12 weeks. Kamal ho gaya na?' 'Kamal aap kar rahe the, yeh toh normal hai!'

7. The player

Shishir had it all. A charming wife, lovely kids, gaadi-bungla and as the brain behind the strategies of a cement company that was spreading its wings all across India, he had the ultimate luxury, the luxury of time. 'Come anytime, go anytime, no problem, but when there is kaam, don't go home, no problem there too.' His main problem in life had been that he felt he would either get a bitch or a brain-dead woman for a wife, but now that his had turned out to be a goddess — adopting a daughter after bearing a biological son, working on the Clean Ganga campaign, stashing his black and white carefully, driving the car herself, etc. — he felt in a good enough position to crack his other problem: weight! More specifically, his paunch. 'And I play tennis, like all the time, but still why?'

One of the necessities of his small town life, he told me, was going to the club / gymkhana. 'Half because there is no entertainment and half because without my carefully planted networks in the club, I would have no money left for entertainment.' He started playing tennis at 33, as that's what the MoS, the quarry owner, the DIG, the who's who of the town were playing. He doesn't remember when this 'compulsion' turned to passion, but now he played for the love of the game and others played for the love of what strings he could pull for them. 'Now I am 36; by 40 I want to break into the national league and get a ranking, just look at Sachin Tendulkar!'

His diet history is actually quite a story but short mein bolu toh, he had given up eating real food for protein shakes with fibre in them to 'lose weight'. 'You will lose games and not weight when you give up real food,' I told him. Anyway the diet was in order soon, no more living off shakes, instead living on real food and supplementing with real protein shake, not the fibre-wala weight-loss type shakes. But then he wrote down his workout recall for me:

Original workout recall:
Every day is the same thing, but since you insist, here goes:
6.30 a.m. to 9:00 a.m. daily play tennis
First 30 mins rounds of tennis courts, with some stretching. Then play game, always tell marker to hit me really difficult shots and really make me run around the court. And then 8.20 to 8.30 a.m. some stretching where my trainer picks up my foot and puts it on his shoulder and I stand in front of him, kya stretch milta hai! And then go to the gym and use the twister, 25 times right, 25 times left and then seated twister same 25 times right, 25 times left.
No change, every day of the week same thing, only if something

really crucial comes up like PTA or something then I bunk and of course travailing.

Analysis:

For starters, tennis, i.e. good, competitive tennis or even state-level tennis, will have players that are highly skilled and with movements so fast that most of the energy generated for the game / practice is produced anaerobically. Refer table on page 37. Now in recreational tennis, which is slower, and where players don't have the same level of skill, even though they wear the clothes, shoes and bands on various body parts like knee, wrist, head, etc., most of the energy is produced aerobically, and therefore with very little after-burn. That's exactly why 3 or even 30 years of recreational tennis will not let you break into any kind of league, forget breaking into the national league. And that's also why all the tennis playing uncles, even the 'regular' ones, have paunches and all.

A 30-minute run is aerobic in nature and if you want your marker to hit you the hard shots, it means you want to enter the anaerobic zone, so for starters you are not following the specificity principle of a warm-up. A 30-minute aerobic warm-up, if anything, eats into the glycogen stores, the fuel that your anaerobic energy uses exclusively. On a low glycogen tank, when you tell the marker to hit hard, he basically only pretends to send across some tough volleys. When you are real competition for the marker, you don't have to beg him for toughness, you have to beg him for forgiveness.

Also, this kind of stretching, with your leg on someone else's shoulder while you stand on the other foot, puts your back into a super awkward position and chances are that you will just snap the hamstring one day. Hamstrings should be stretched, not snapped. And for heaven's sake, vigorous shaking or movements on the twister don't 'release' the back; if anything they just jam it. And post the game when the back is already tired (ya baba, you run with the legs but the spine and the muscles around it are involved very much), twisting it mercilessly is, for the lack of better word, cruel.

A good stretch, be it for the hamstrings or for the back, doesn't need 25 reps on each side or any vigorous movements. A nice, slow stretch, repeated 2-3 times on each side, more than releases any tension in the muscle. Also we must remember that we have more than a hamstring and a back in our body — there's the neck, the shoulder, the quads, the arms, so your stretching program must involve each of these body parts too.

One can take the game of a racquet sport to the next level only when you train your body anaerobically. Strength train in the gym, build a good stretching program and maintain specificity of the warm up / cool down to the actual game. Basically it needs much more than just showing up daily at the court and playing. Though I must say that this works when your age is in single digits, 6 to 9, and in most cases even when you add 1 in front of that single digit. Start them early, watch them grow and don't seek to bask in their glory (here I mean your children), and teach them to play for the love of the sport.

Modified workout plan:

Anyway, my guy was a CA, sharp in the brain, and understood aerobic and anaerobic as different countries and the fuels that they use as their currencies. And just like different countries use specific currencies, certain games will need higher amount or development of certain energy systems and therefore different fuels. He decided that more of his week should be dedicated to staying and producing energy in the anaerobic zone, so here's the workout he planned himself after all the gyan.

	Exercise Plan	**Remarks**
Day 1	Lower body strength training	Anaerobic
Day 2	Rest	NA
Day 3	LT (Running/Cycling)	Lactate threshold
Day 4	Tennis Day	Aerobic
Day 5	Upper body strength training	Anaerobic
Day 6	Rest	NA
Day 7	Tennis Day	Aerobic

From playing tennis twice a week, he slowly graduated to playing thrice in about 12 weeks as he made gains in strength and speed and dropped some body fat and his game dramatically improved too. He quit on twisters and learnt some core stability exercises and stretches and performed them on the rest days. His following increased, this time even for weight loss tips ;).

Extras

1. The doctor–trainer–dietician lafda

Ideally these three should be keeping you, your comfort and your wellbeing as their main agenda, but that is not how it often turns out.

Your doctor is clueless about exercise science but is either too proud or too ignorant to admit that. He / she however leaves no stone unturned to get you off whatever little exercise you may be doing, other than a walk of course (Bharat ko raaj). And since every advice is offered after treating you like the most useless entity on earth — makes you wait endlessly, clueless about your name, barely looks up from the desk or prescription or blood report while talking at you, never gives you a chance to speak, etc. — you take it with the seriousness of a boy scout who Obama just shook hands with. In our heads he / she is 'educated', 'very famous', 'has no time', 'long waiting queue' and other such factors which therefore make his statements like 'don't bend, don't lift, don't move' sound like some aakashvani preventing us from further discomfort than what we already are in.

The dietician gives you similar treatment, just that the waiting time is shorter and so is your gratitude in return, but you get pulled up for not 'following' the diet, and are given 2 sheets full of foods you must avoid. Your heart sinks and you are clueless about what CAN you finally eat if you must avoid banana, chikoo, mango, rice, dal, ghee, etc. Of course, no exercise, surely no weight training or asanas, but pranayama is ok and yes, walk. Everybody please walk. She is clueless about exercise science too and is stuck in a time machine and still counts calories and says things like — if calorie in is less than calorie out then there's weight loss. Yay!! Anyway we are only happy to meet them and follow their advice coz it's in tune with what we read every day in the papers and what the doctor confirms: a) everything that your family and forefathers have been doing is wrong and b) Ghee, rice, sugar, etc. are your enemy, preferably give up on milk also, if not switch to skim milk.

The trainer here is the person who spends maximum time with you, often waiting for you to show up in the gym, knows your name, where you holidayed last summer, how that back issue or BP even came about, remembers your child's roll number too. But he is on the fringes of an upcoming profession, either belongs to the middle or the lower middle class, hasn't really studied beyond 10th or 12th and can barely speak English. So he / she may know why you should do weight training, why weights will help you lower resting BP, how it leads to better glucose uptake by cells, how the doctor is taking the wrong approach with you, why you should bother more about sugar spikes and drops in the day versus your PP and fasting values, but ask them to put those things in words and they mess up! And how!

Anyway, the feudal system that we belong to respects education, class, English-speaking abilities (not necessary in this order though) much more than genuine concern for us. So who loses in the end? The trainer? No, they move on to another client, the doctor always has the next patient waiting and the dietician has a talk to give in a rotary. The loser in this lafda is you. The clueless 'patient', 'client', whatever you call yourself, who gets tugged in opposite directions by people you trust your health with.

Ideally this is what should happen: your doctor should ask you to work out and not share his opinion about what you should not do, you should also understand that he is in no position to offer advice on exercise. Your dietician should outgrow this 'calorie in, calorie out and what works for the West is applicable in my country too' approach. The trainer should get educated and instead of flexing his bicep in front of the mirror, should flex his talking prowess. And you, my dear, should know that health is not built by 'professionals' but by the person who resides in the body.

You want to look better, feel fitter, then you should be in charge. Look after yourself and take decisions, medical or otherwise, out of love and not out of fear. The natural tendency of the human soul is growth and expansion, so to stay true to your nature you should be able to do more with your body as you age, not less. Anyway, it is not so black and white; not all trainers are good at what they do, not all doctors are ignorant and not all dieticians are stuck up. The newer, younger breed is surely changing, feeling more comfy in their skin than what they ever were. There really is nothing like having the doctor, dietician and trainer on the same page, it accelerates your recovery, wipes out the memory of past pain, fills you with optimism, with the hope of a brighter, better, healthier future and most importantly gives the control of your health in your hands. No one's scaring you and no one's talking mumbo-jumbo to you. The doctor–dietician–trainer trio exists for your wellbeing and for your seva and samadhan, not the other way round, never!

2. Learn to unhear

Long ago, in 2004 to be precise, I was training one of my 'famous' clients, doing some uphill running on Altamount Road. We were the only two running uphill, dodging the 'morning walkers' when someone shouted, 'Gadhedo bau fast bhagheche.' As soon as I heard these words uttered, my temper flew and I did what every Mumbai girl does, turned around and gave khunnas. It was met with murmured laughter and then finally there was silence. I ran ahead, turned back one more time and gave some more khunnas, it was met with some more silence, heads went down and the fat snobs of Altamount Road walked uphill in their white shorts and tees over flawless paunches.

With the snobs gone, I had to turn my rage on someone else so now it was going to be my clients's turn. It was our uphill day and till I met these 'morning walkers' I was on a high. My runner hadn't once slouched on the uphill, had landed perfectly without jarring his joints, from a heel striker, he was turning to a mid-foot striker, the weather wasn't humid and sultry, it was just perfect and I should have been happy. I was anything but.

As we got into post run stretching, my client asked, 'Come on, why are you so angry?' 'Because you are not,' I answered. 'And why should I be angry,' he asked. 'Because you heard everything they said,' and I crossed my arms and moved away. 'What did they say?' 'Come on, I know you heard.' 'Yes I did. Pahili vaar ladki aane peeche daudis, opposite hoye. Saala Mercedes ne BMW park karkich, par gadhedo bau fast bhageche.

'But RD, when you hear things, you must know what to make of them and what is relevant. Aren't you thrilled that even they noticed that I am running faster? We have been training since July, it's only October and random people can see that I am faster, we should be celebrating and you are wasting time feeling angry. You are so angry that you asked me to stop running earlier than usual, no feedback on running and now no attention to the fact that I am cheating while stretching my hamstrings.

'If you must overhear conversation that is not meant for you, then you MUST know what to hear and what to unhear.' This then has become my founding philosophy in the gym and other exercise places or at social outings where bodies, workouts, diets and trainers invariably get discussed. And here are some examples of how you can unhear and only hear what you should:

What is said	What you should hear
She is hardly size zero but she's bloody fit.	She's bloody fit.
She's so regular in the gym, must have a very caring husband.	She's very regular in the gym.
Look at that paunch but she has the confidence to carry off that skimpy thing.	She has the confidence to carry off anything.
You have such a beautiful face, you will look so much prettier if you lose some weight.	You have such a beautiful face, so pretty!

He's constantly looking at himself in the mirror after he has gotten regular at the gym.	He has gotten regular in the gym.
Will always sleep till late but if it's cricket / football, etc., will bloody wake up at 5 a.m.	He is commited to his game.
Won't eat a thing post dinner even if you beg at her feet.	She's very committed to eating right.

Exercise tracker

Maintain these sheets so that you can keep a track of your workout, spot mistakes and make progress. Maintain the tracker for 12 weeks in a row and it can teach you much more than any fitness guide.

Weight training days

Date	Exercise	Sets	Weights (Lbs Or Kgs)	Repetitions

Cardio days

Date	Exercise	Speed/ Rpm	Incline/ Resistance	Time (Mins)	Distance (Kms)	Rpe

Acknowledgements

This book is conceived and written from the minds of many beautiful people I have met and from conversations, heard and overheard, in gyms, on treks, trains, coffee shops, weddings and funerals and of course on my Facebook and Twitter pages. But then in acknowledgements I can only thank people whose names I know and who know that they have helped me immensely. So here goes, in no order of preference:

- To the city of Mumbai, which allows people like me, non-mainstream people, to make a living and live with dignity.
- For my family and friends for wholeheartedly supporting every venture I undertake, including book writing.
- My clients for doing my naam roshan in every possible way. I really do owe everything to you.
- My many trainer friends for the stories and gym kahanis, advice and sharing of routines and most importantly for teaching me both what to do and not do, with everything from training to watches, hairstyles and finances.
- The doctors who work with my clients for keeping their caution aside and being not just ok but encouraging exercise.
- My team for always covering up for me.
- Deepthi and everyone at Westland for their patience.
- GP, without whom no book of mine can ever be written.
- My yoga teachers: the late Karin O-Bannon, Zubin Zarthoshtimanesh, Kobad Variava and Usha Devi of

Rishikesh for their patient, kind and compassionate teaching.

- Siddhartha Krishna of Omkarananda ashram and Swami Govindananda of the Sivananda lineage for their teachings of philosophy in practice.
- And finally, huge thanks to you; it's the readers who make a book, not writers, publishers and marketers.